I0558507

Dr. Martinelli's Vision & Neurology Casebook

Real World Insights for Primary Eye Care & Family Medicine

The Fine Art of Patient Management

John R Martinelli MD OD FAAO

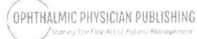
OPHTHALMIC PHYSICIAN PUBLISHING
Sharing the Fine Art of Patient Management

To Melissa...
These pages would not exist without you.
Thank you for always being there.
You are my forever.
XO

Contents

Medical Disclaimer

Please note the information contained within this book is for educational purposes only. All effort has been executed to present accurate, up-to-date, reliable, complete information. The content within this book has been derived from various sources. Please consult a licensed physician before implementing diagnostic methods and/or treatments outlined in this book.

By reading this book, the reader agrees that under no circumstances is the author responsible for any losses, direct or indirect, that are incurred because of the use of the information contained within this book, including, but not limited to, errors, omissions, or inaccuracies.

Please note the information provided below is for general informational purposes. It is not intended to diagnose, treat, cure, or prevent any disease, and it should not be relied upon as a substitute for consultations with qualified healthcare professionals.

Medical Disclaimer

Ophthalmic Physician Publishing strives to ensure the information presented is accurate and up to date, but we make no representations or warranties of any kind, express or implied, about the completeness, accuracy, reliability, suitability, or availability with respect to the information provided. Any reliance you place on such information is strictly at your own risk.

———

Foreword

James L. Fanelli, OD, FAAO

Great health care providers continually strive to improve their knowledge base by learning from past patient encounters and medical knowledge, to provide better patient outcomes for future patient encounters. While striving to expand our knowledge as health care providers is a must, having the proper resources to refer to is critical, especially when it comes to neuro-ophthalmic disorders. There are many pieces to this clinically challenging area of healthcare, and having a reference guide to help navigate these sometimes life and vision threatening cases is invaluable.

This is a fantastic guide for busy clinicians in the trenches who encounter a disease process where all the pieces sometimes don't necessarily fit together or are simply complex in nature. With a system wide approach to various eye diseases, Dr. Martinelli has succinctly and expertly summarized the salient points related to normal anatomic structure and physiologic processes, and beautifully lays out the underlying abnormal process.

The clues that present in the clinical scenario of a patient visit help guide each of us along a path of a problem focused examination, ultimately leading to an appropriate diagnosis and management plan. Having pertinent, thought-provoking differential diagnoses, as well as discussing nuances of the cases, Dr. Martinelli not only organizes the clinical information relevant to the case at hand, but also lays the foundation for the thought processes needed to manage similar, yet fundamentally different cases. All in an organized, intuitive manner.

Hippocrates wrote: Whenever the art of medicine is loved, there is also a love of humanity. Dr. Martinelli clearly loves medicine, and his creation of this book for all of us knee deep in clinical care shows his love for humanity, by helping all of us to be better deliverers of care.

Every eye care provider and general practitioner needs this book!

James L. Fanelli, OD, FAAO
Optometric Physician
Cape Fear Eye Associates
Wilmington, NC

Edward C. Kondrot, MD

This is a very important book all general physicians and eye doctors should read and study. Neurologic diseases are often life-threatening, and when first presenting as a vision problem, it is important for doctors to quickly make the correct diagnosis.

Dr. Martinelli takes the complex world of neuro-ophthalmology and presents cases that are often misdiagnosed even by seasoned practitioners. He adds and discusses various differential diagnoses with sections dedicated to "thinking deeper", helping you become a more critical thinker.

Each case is summarized with learning points as well as questions and answers. Studying the cases Dr. Martinelli presents will help you grow as a better clinician by becoming more comfortable recognizing sight and life-threatening neurologic problems. Many of his examples will most certainly present in your practice.

Edward C. Kondrot, MD
Board Certified Ophthalmologist
Pittsburgh, PA

Colby M. Genrich, MD

In Dr. Martinelli's unique casebook, readers will find an immersive narrative into often mysterious neuro-ophthalmic diagnoses and management.

Through real-world everyday patients, this book quickly moves past traditional textbooks demonstrating a process of reasoning and decision making backed by clinical experience. The clinical scenarios are representative of what we often encounter in daily practice, which need to be first managed on the front lines in primary care. Reading through the cases, physicians and medical professionals will find genuine examples in the practice of treating the whole patient.

Recent research underscores the efficacy of case-based teaching methodologies in medical education, solidifying its role in fostering critical thinking, clinical reasoning, and problem-solving skills among students and clinicians (Gasim 2024). Grounded in practical medical teaching, "Dr. Martinelli's Vision & Neurology Casebook" is a fresh and creative take to medical education.

Dr. Martinelli breaks down each case into manageable and discussion-ready segments, perfect for small roundtable discussions or lecture hall and team-based learning environments. By integrating theory with practical application, this book helps support medical professionals with an additional resource necessary to navigate the complexities of real-world medicine with confidence and competence.

Colby M. Genrich, MD, CAQSM
Assistant Professor, Family Medicine Clerkship Director, Sports Medicine Fellowship Program Director, Texas Tech University – Paul L. Foster School of Medicine

Zsofia Szabo, MD, MS

Dr. Martinelli's Vision & Neurology Casebook: Real World Insights for Primary Eye Care and Family Medicine is an insightful and well structured clinical-vignette based approach to help master fundamental understanding of basic neuro-ophthalmic disease and conditions.

His clinical pearls are engaging, and the overall tone of the book is comfortable and easy to follow. It is a refreshing take on the often intimidating and challenging complexity of neuro-ophthalmic disease, tackling the subject without overly complicated pathophysiology, thus making it a useful practical guide. It is an excellent resource for beginners, as well as for those who wish to refresh their knowledge.

Rather than having to review dense comprehensive textbooks, which are burdened with extensive technicality, the substantial information here is presented in concise, unpretentious, and easily understandable terms. Dr. Martinelli's bread and butter, as well as caviar cases highlight how to approach clinical problems with classic examples that will help commit concepts to memory and increase learning efficiency.

Zsofia Szabo MD, MS
Board Certified Neurologist
Sarasota Memorial Hospital
Sarasota, FL

Michael Aidi, MD

Dr. Martinelli's *Vision & Neurology Casebook* goes where few have gone.

Through well-written and more importantly easily readable comprehensible and instructive cases, your confidence can build to take on similar cases under real-world conditions. Dr. Martinelli also elaborates on the pharmacological treatment of certain conditions with dosages which, in particular, is where many others fall short.

You will appreciate the laid-back, almost colloquial or conversational style of the book as opposed to a traditional textbook. The pages fly by as you feel more like you're discussing the case with a colleague rather than referencing a text, allowing you to absorb more of the information than you realize.

This material has come straight from the mind of a clinician who has experienced it, and ingrained it after 36 years of practice. The details are there, but you won't be bogged down by them so to more easily see the forest through the trees.

Michael Aidi, MD
Board Certified Neuroradiologist
Baptist Health Memorial Hospital
Boca Raton, FL

Introduction to The Fine Art of Patient Management

John R Martinelli

Imagine If...

A Patient in Your Chair...

A new patient, a 36-year-old gentleman with a past medical history of hypertension, comes to see you with recent diplopia progressively worsening over the previous week.

He initially visited his long-time optometrist who performed a comprehensive examination, including dilation and a peripheral retinal exam, finally attributed his symptoms to possibly high blood pressure and advised him to see his primary care physician (PCP).

A couple days later, he went to his PCP's office, where a Physician Assistant (PA) evaluated him without the physician present. The PA then referred him to you citing "just" double vision when speaking to your staff by telephone.

When you saw him, he presented with true progressive diplopia which was characteristic of a fourth nerve (IVn) palsy of his left eye. His diplopia had also worsened since the initial onset and was now constant and oblique.

Recognizing the urgency, you send him immediately to the emergency department (ED) with a note outlining his clinical presentation and requesting stroke protocol with neurology consult. You know the constant and progressive nature is ominous supporting a potential space occupying source.

Upon arrival to the ED, the staff seemed surprised by him being sent so urgently without additional signs or symptoms. Vitals were normal, CT head was unremarkable, told "everything is fine" and discharged. He was asked to follow-up again with his eye doctor – which is where he started.

Unfortunately, this is not an *"imagine if"* scenario but is real life - an example of a not uncommon referral merry-go-round.

Does this pattern suggest a lack of competency, inadequate care coordination, and/or communication breakdown? Could it be simply no one else is prepared to share responsibility?

It is frustrating to witness such lapses in care and is a big part of my motivation for this book and series. My hope is to encourage you to be the best you can be for your patients - to become confident by gaining knowledge and experience, creating the power to assume full responsibility for each of them.

A Journey in Philosophy

Vision & Neurology Casebook is the first in my systems-based series of clinical publications, marking the culmination of a personal journey that began with a very modest act of writing several years ago.

My promise is to demonstrate the means to positively impact and grow your practice internally, directly through your patients, exemplified by real world clinical scenarios. Understanding how and why critical thinking leads to problem-solving, mixed with expertise in communication, is crucial in providing superior care and guidance for your patients and practice development.

I emphasize the importance of learning to fully communicate one-on-one with your patients empathetically and with truthfulness. This is essential above all things. Ultimately, your expertise and care can only be as effective as your genuine and personal connection in this way. You will invariably keep your patients with you where they belong, as well as their families, friends, and everyone else creating perpetual referrals for a lifetime. They won't need or want to go anywhere else!

These daily opportunities to begin a relationship with your patients are achieved by learning to place yourself on their level, learning to speak their language whether they are 9 years old or 99 years old. In turn, they will provide you with limitless professional and personal growth bringing you closer to this illusive concept of what success really is.

The series is based on my extensive written case discussions from personal experience, laying emphasis on teaching ophthalmic medicine as it relates to general medicine. Presented in a practical way to benefit your patients, I believe these discussions will help lead the way for you to also create and grow a successful practice for the right reasons—founded completely in primary care with the "*Patient in Your Chair*" front and center.

On a personal note, this journey came to be amidst close family tragedies. I unexpectedly discovered a form of therapy in the act of writing and sharing my many interesting patient encounters to my private social media group, for anyone who might be interested. It also became a constructive way to continue studying and learning by putting down my thought process on paper in often complicated daily clinical scenarios.

Over time, I began to realize the path I was on also evolved into a reflective exploration of not only my professional experience, but very much personally in terms of recognizing and appreciating what is most important to continue to grow a practice of great success. It became a time of important reminders and exercises in *philosophy*.

Let's remember we must first understand people. Then learning to believe and live by a philosophy they are the priority, not you or me. An unselfish philosophy which is centered around taking personal responsibility for the care of people, who also happen to be our patients, and with complete total honesty. Success begins here, and we practice it with our ears, what's in between, as well as how, when, and what we speak.

Fast forward to a period of more than seven years of steady writing, I found I had compiled countless teaching points and learning opportunities purely by writing down many of my everyday patient experiences. A wealth of clinical scenarios I have also painstakingly categorized by organ system, for which I'm thrilled to have the opportunity to share.

The Art of it All

Like many of us in the medical field, I share an obsession and fascination with finding solutions to problems. Seeing and feeling the appreciation of so many of my patients over the years, knowing I'm doing what I should be doing, has become my driving force leading this humble attempt to also teach others.

What you'll find here are solutions and answers to clinical questions I'm asking myself during the day, as I strive to do the right things the right way and for the right reasons. In essence, it is thinking out loud for what I like to call thought-based medicine in eye care. Therefore, you will not find academic references anywhere within these pages. I go beyond textbooks and classrooms, attempting to demonstrate a certain wisdom that can only be found through daily real-life patient interactions.

Clinical practice enhances our problem-solving abilities and grows our instincts, which cannot be easily verbalized or even explained. The ability to discern even the subtlest nuances affecting an individual's well-being is a talent that can only be developed through continuous exposure to the many unique individuals in our chair every single day – over years. What we do is truly an art.

In addition to a philosophy of patient care, my goal is to provide you with an additional resource when encountering some common and perhaps not so common conditions when the puzzle pieces just don't fit together. To help guide you through a clinical journey by unlocking pertinent ocular dilemmas and mysteries with select cases.

I'm certain these important but sometimes forgotten medical principles will elevate your own personal journey encompassing vision preservation, life enhancement, and on occasion, life-saving interventions.

How to Learn from This Book

Cases are organized based on an individual's presenting signs and/or symptoms, just the same as encountering patients in daily practice.

With each clinical scenario presented, you will first need to think through the case and consider a series of key questions to determine an appropriate workup, diagnosis, and management. This will help guide your rationale to methodically work through your approach.

When you see **"*Think Deeper!*"** ask yourself the following questions:

- **What are my differential diagnoses?** Attempt to formulate at least three differential diagnoses. What is the rationale for each diagnosis on your list? Why exactly is one differential more likely than another?
- **What is my top differential?** What is your most powerful rationale for it to be most likely? Be reminded a top differential is not necessarily the final definitive diagnosis.
- **Do I understand my full role in primary care?** Unnecessary referrals and defensive medicine are no way to practice, not to mention a disservice to the individual who can often be taken care of within your legal scope of practice.

- **What investigations can I do in-house?** Are you positioned to manage your patient in-office? Also consider outside labs and imaging you can order. What is justified and supported by your evaluation and what might be a waste of resources? Remember, all diagnostics must change or influence your management - there is no such thing as "routine" testing, labs, and/or imaging!
- **Can I wear different hats?** Think deeper regarding diagnostics, labs, and imaging beyond primary care. Put your sub-specialty hat on. Learn to understand expanded management which might be required to solve your patients' problems. Don't hesitate to order those investigations to guide your patient accordingly.
- **What are my next steps in management?** Will you solely treat and manage your patient? Will you refer on? If your patient is not managed and handled properly, including a lack of truly listening and communicating effectively, are there potential medical and/or legal issues which can be of consequence?
- **What are my learning opportunities?** Think deeper and be honest with yourself regarding real-life understanding with respect to the pathophysiology of each differential. Study. Every patient in your chair also happens to be your #1 learning opportunity over and above anything else.
- **Do I practice empathy?** Can you imagine yourself as the patient? Are you conscious of discussing your thoughts and differentials empathetically? We must remember it is a real person, not a clinical case in a textbook. And if working with a distraught or angry

individual, are you skilled in "the fine art of verbal anesthesia"? We also practice psychology daily, perhaps more so than anything!

Consider these questions before reading the discussion and management section of the case, you should then have a top diagnosis and plan in mind. Envision your bedside manner, rapport, tone, and how you will relate one-on-one. I believe these qualities contribute more strongly to your patients' well-being versus immediately solving their clinical puzzle.

Remember, in medicine nothing is black and white. There are shades of gray, no rules, and above all assume nothing! Each of us have different approaches to managing patients, however, in the hands of competency our results will often be the same.

Finally, study your working diagnosis. Master it. Including risk factors, diagnostic criteria, incidence, prevalence, management options, and additional pertinent concepts. Legitimate evidence-based medicine is strongest when it is from your own experience. General medicine as well as those of us in primary eye care must pursue expansive knowledge and concepts across all specialties.

Going Forward

Throughout this book you will find:

- **Clinical Scenarios**: A diverse array of real-life patients, our true teachers giving us opportunities to master the dynamics of primary eye care and medicine.

- *A "Think Deeper"* **Philosophy**: Critical thinking and thought-based medicine refining diagnostic precision.
- **High-Yield Discussion & Management**: Focused on practical knowledge and the distilled wisdom of real-world private practice, leaving behind textbook jargon.
- **Differential Diagnoses & Medical Rationale**: Scrutinizing the clinical scenario with "assume nothing" possibilities.
- **Learning Points**: Sharing observations and philosophies in the art of thoughtful patient care.
- **Questions & Answers**: Test your understanding of key concepts specific to each clinical scenario.

We must always be equipped to make a positive impact in our patients' lives. This is why we are out there on the front lines in daily practice, and why we should continue to study hard to do what we do. This is why it's called *practice*. And it never stops! Let's not forget it's all about people, our patients.

However, it's also important to appreciate your patients make a conscious choice to see you and not the doctor across town. Why is this? Why do they choose you? I hope this book series will help you become the first choice in your community leading to a form of success beyond anything you ever anticipated or imagined.

And as you also strive to master this elusive art of medicine and patient care, a certain wisdom will find its way to you. A wisdom, for which you and I are fortunate to share in taking care of people.

John R. Martinelli
June 16, 2024

MUSCLE, NERVE, *or* BRAIN?

Larry Gray, OD
Pennsylvania College of Optometry
Philadelphia, PA

Section 1

Muscle

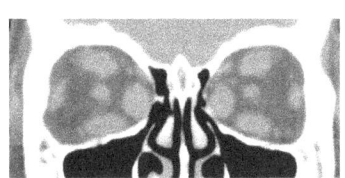

"Neuromuscular diseases reveal the incredible intricacy and resilience of the human body, pushing us to find new ways to support and heal".

– Dr. Stanley Appel

Eye Won't Wake Up

History of Present Illness (HPI)

A 78-year-old lady is in your chair. For the last several months, she has had trouble opening her left eye when she wakes up in the morning. However, when she rubs it, after a couple of minutes it becomes easier to open and goes back to normal.

Review of Systems (ROS)

She has had no recent change in vision, loss of vision, diplopia, or pain. She sometimes notices her lid also droops during the day. No symptoms of dry eye or discharge. No recent weight loss, fever, or night sweats. Occasionally, she experiences mild neck discomfort.

Past Medical History (PMH)

Hypothyroidism and iron deficiency anemia. Anxiety and depression over many years. A lipoma in her neck was discovered during her last physical exam.

Family History (FH)

Her parents both had a history of cardiovascular disease, hypertension, and diabetes.

Medications and Allergies

She takes levothyroxine 75 mcg, sertraline 50 mg daily, and iron supplements. She has no known allergies to medications, foods, or environmental factors.

Ophthalmic Examination

- **Best Corrected Visual Acuity (BCVA):** 20/25 OD, 20/30 OS.
- **Pupils:** Pupils equal, round, reactive to light and accommodation, no afferent pupillary defect. PERRLA (-)APD
- **Extraocular Muscles (EOMs):** Full, without diplopia.
- **Visual Field (VF):** Full OU.
- **Intraocular Pressure (IOP):** 19 OD, 20 OS.
- **Anterior Segment:** Clear cornea, quiet and deep anterior chamber, pseudophakic with nicely placed posterior chamber IOL's OU.
- **Posterior Segment:** Optic disc, macula, vessels,

vitreous, retina unremarkable OU. Trace macular drusen and pigment mottling OU.

- **Eyelids:** Dermatochalasis OU, with ptosis OS.
- **Optical Coherence Tomography (OCT):** Normal optic nerve and retinal nerve fiber layer (rNFL) OU, macula with early drusen and RPE changes OU. No evidence of disc edema OU.

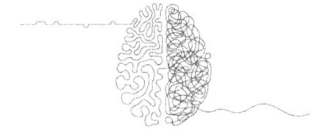

Think Deeper!

Discussion and Management

Her difficulty opening her left eye in the mornings, as well as transient ptosis during the day, brings to your mind multiple possible sources and scenarios.

You consider myasthenia gravis (MG), particularly ocular myasthenia, which can manifest as progressive muscle weakness worsening with fatigue or toward the end of the day. In her case, early morning fatigue with ptosis noticed during the day may be your first clue. The improvement in ptosis after rubbing her eye suggests a mechanical enhancement of neuromuscular transmission, supporting an etiology of myasthenia.

Your diagnostic investigations should involve specific labs for confirmation, and to rule-out other potential sources. Labs targeting acetylcholine receptor antibodies (AChRAb) is your top priority, as their presence is highly specific for myasthenia gravis. These include binding antibodies, which are the most commonly detected, blocking antibodies that interfere with acetylcholine binding, and modulating antibodies that alter the number of acetylcholine receptors and their functions on the muscle surface. When AChR antibodies are not detected, labs for muscle-specific kinase (MuSK) antibodies become key in diagnosing seronegative myasthenia gravis.

Electromyography (EMG) is also an important diagnostic tool. Repetitive nerve stimulation measures the electrical response of muscles to repeated nerve stimulation, where a decremental response indicates myasthenia gravis. Single-fiber EMG, a more sensitive test, detects abnormalities in neuromuscular transmission providing further confirmation.

The edrophonium test, also known as the tensilon test, involves administering IV edrophonium which temporarily improves muscle function in individuals with myasthenia by inhibiting acetylcholinesterase. This increases the availability of acetylcholine leading to improved neuromuscular response. This improvement following administration also supports the diagnosis. The tensilon test is not utilized as it once was due to high false positives, and the development of serologic antibody testing.

Another simple but effective test is the ice pack test. With ptosis, applying an ice pack to the eyelid for a few minutes can temporarily yield improvement, suggesting myasthenia. This is because the transmission of acetylcholine is improved at cooler temperatures.

There is an association between myasthenia gravis and thyroid disorders such as Hashimoto's thyroiditis, the most common cause of hypothyroidism in the U.S. and in regions with inadequate iodine intake. This association is not surprising considering both have an autoimmune basis. In Hashimoto's thyroiditis, antibodies target the thyroid gland which includes anti-thyroid peroxidase (anti-TPO) antibodies and anti-thyroglobulin antibodies. These antibodies trigger chronic inflammation and progressive destruction of thyroid tissue over time. Initially creating a hyperthyroid state, then euthyroid, and ultimately hypothyroidism over a period of years. However, anti-TPO and anti-thyroglobulin antibodies are rarely investigated when an individual presents in an already hypothyroid state, as the treatment is the same despite the etiology via lifetime thyroid hormone replacement therapy.

In her case, being treated with levothyroxine you already know she has become hypothyroid, which in fact is the end result of Hashimoto's. Therefore, obtaining anti-TPO labs may in fact confirm Hashimoto's which will help complete her clinical picture. Additionally, since myasthenia gravis can be associated with various autoimmune conditions, other labs such as ANA and rheumatoid factor can be pursued if clinically indicated.

In your work-up, chest imaging via CT or MRI should also be performed looking for thymoma, as there is a known association between thymoma and myasthenia gravis. A thymoma is an immune-dysfunctional mass originating from epithelial cells of the thymus, located in the anterior mediastinum. The thymus plays a crucial role in the development of the immune system, particularly during childhood as it is involved in the maturation of T-lymphocytes (T-cells) which are essential for adaptive immunity.

Given her history of a neck lipoma, you also consider Horner's syndrome, which results from disruption of sympathetic pathways. The classic triad of ptosis, miosis, and anhidrosis is a thought, however, she does not have a miotic pupil. If indicated, imaging studies including MRI or CT of the neck, cervical spine, and chest may help identify any compressive lesions affecting the sympathetic chain.

Your management of her condition will depend on the underlying diagnosis. If myasthenia gravis is confirmed, initial treatment with cholinesterase inhibitors such as pyridostigmine may be effective. Immunosuppressive therapy, including corticosteroids, may be necessary for more severe cases. In the case of a confirmed thymoma, surgical excision would be indicated.

Finally, if ocular myasthenia is confirmed, you emphasize the importance of adhering to treatment and recognizing signs of potential complications. Specifically respiratory difficulties, which can occur with generalized myasthenia gravis.

Differential Diagnoses and Rationale

- **Ocular Myasthenia Gravis:** Fluctuating ptosis progressing as the day goes on, and if improvement with rest suggest neuromuscular junction involvement. Diagnostic confirmation through anti-acetylcholine receptor antibody testing, repetitive nerve stimulation, and single-fiber electromyography is necessary.
- **Horner's Syndrome:** Considered due to the presence of ptosis and a neck mass, which may have been

incorrectly "assumed" to be a lipoma. However, signs such as miosis and anhidrosis are lacking, pointing away from this diagnosis. Imaging studies of the neck and chest can help identify any compressive lesions affecting the sympathetic chain.

- **Thymoma:** Associated with myasthenia gravis and requires evaluation via chest imaging. Although more common in younger patients, it can present in older adults and should not be dismissed.
- **Compressive Orbital Mass Lesion:** Lipoma or other mass creating mechanical compression, though less likely given the transient nature of her signs and symptoms and the isolated ptosis.

Learning Points

- Understand the pathophysiology of myasthenia gravis and its presentation, particularly ocular myasthenia, characterized by fluctuating muscle weakness with ptosis worsening as the day goes on.
- Recognize the importance of a comprehensive neuro-ophthalmic evaluation to rule out other potential causes of ptosis, including Horner's syndrome.
- Emphasize the role of imaging studies in identifying compressive lesions or masses that which can contribute to ptosis.
- Highlight the necessity of patient education, particularly potential respiratory difficulties, with regular follow-up for treatment response and to adjust management strategies as needed.

Questions

What are key diagnostic investigations for confirming myasthenia gravis?

Anti-acetylcholine receptor antibody and MuSK labs, repetitive nerve stimulation studies, and single-fiber electromyography (SFEMG).

How can Horner's syndrome be differentiated from other etiologies of ptosis?

Horner's syndrome can be differentiated by the presence of the classic triad of ptosis, miosis, and anhidrosis. Imaging studies such as MRI or CT of the neck and chest can help identify any compressive lesions affecting the sympathetic chain.

What is the significance of a chest CT with suspected myasthenia gravis?

A chest CT is necessary for individuals with suspected or confirmed myasthenia gravis to evaluate for thymoma, which is commonly associated with myasthenia gravis. Thymoma can present in both younger and older adults and requires surgical excision if confirmed.

Disney Double

History of Present Illness (HPI)

A 39-year-old gentleman is in your chair with recent onset of varying diplopia and severe peri-orbital pain, peaking at an intensity of 10 out of 10. His symptoms started about one month prior to seeing you, after sustaining a right foot and ankle injury when he tripped and fell running with his daughter at Disney World in Orlando, Florida. He has no previous history of ocular or vision problems.

Review of Systems (ROS)

In addition to his diplopia and ocular pain, he developed an erythematous, edematous, and tender dermatitis above his ankle shortly after he fell. He denies nausea, vomiting, headaches, or sensory deficits, but has continuous pain in his leg when walking since this occurred.

Past Medical History (PMH)

Type-2 diabetes with borderline control and osteogenesis imperfecta type-1.

Family History (FH)

Father and mother with type-2 diabetes and hypertension.

Medications and Allergies

Metformin 500 mg twice daily and a daily bisphosphonate. He has no known allergies to medications, foods, or environmental factors.

Ophthalmic Examination

- **Best Corrected Visual Acuity (BCVA):** 20/20 OU.
- **Pupils:** Pupils equal, round, responsive to light and accommodation, no afferent pupillary defect. PERRLA, (-)APD.
- **Extraocular Muscles (EOMs):** Non-specific, transient, varying strabismus with diplopia.
- **Visual Field (VF):** Full OU.

- **Intraocular Pressure (IOP):** 15 mmHg OU.
- **Anterior Segment:** Clear cornea, deep and quiet anterior chamber, clear lens OU.
- **Posterior Segment:** Healthy optic disc, macula, vasculature, vitreous, retina OU.
- **Optical Coherence Tomography (OCT):** Normal optic nerve and retinal nerve fiber layer (rNFL) OU, macula clear with good foveal contour OU. No evidence of disc edema OU.
- **Cover Test:** Intermittent exotropia and hypertropia OD, occasionally OS, varying with gaze direction, suggesting a complex and non-specific pattern.

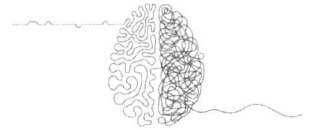

Think Deeper!

Discussion and Management

Your patient proves to be a diagnostic challenge, with varying diplopia and severe ocular pain in the context of recent trauma and a history of chronic medical conditions. His variability in diplopia, coupled with severe pain, suggests a dynamic etiology affecting ocular neuromuscular control. You consider the possibility of transient increasing intracranial pressure, or a waxing and waning inflammatory source within the orbit or cavernous sinus.

You immediately order expanded imaging targeting the orbit, cavernous sinus, brainstem, and cranial nerves. MRI with FIESTA protocol as well as CT angiography is absolutely indicated assessing for vascular anomalies, inflammatory processes, or compressive lesions to explain his presentation. These imaging modalities are crucial to visualize soft tissue structures and vascular components, especially within the orbit and cavernous sinus which are often implicated in complex ocular motility disorders.

Specific vascular etiologies must be carefully considered. Carotid-cavernous fistula (CCF) is an abnormal connection between the carotid artery and the cavernous sinus which can produce increased pressure within the cavernous sinus, affecting the contained cranial nerves creating varying diplopia and severe pain. Symptoms typically include pulsatile tinnitus, proptosis, and conjunctival engorgement. MRI and CT angiography can help identify the presence of a fistula and guide management, which can involve endovascular intervention.

Cavernous sinus thrombosis (CST), although rare, is a condition involving thrombus formation within the cavernous sinus often presenting with severe headache, ocular pain, proptosis, and cranial nerve palsies. Risk factors include infection, trauma, and hypercoagulable states. MRI with venography (MRV) is the imaging modality of choice to detect thrombosis, and prompt anticoagulation therapy is critical to prevent further complications.

Conditions such as Tolosa-Hunt syndrome, an idiopathic inflammatory disorder of the cavernous sinus should also be considered. It presents with painful ophthalmoplegia and is diagnosed primarily through exclusion, supported by imaging findings of inflammation in the cavernous sinus. Corticosteroids are typically the treatment.

Most important in his case, infectious etiologies must also be explored, especially given his history of trauma and the presence of dermatologic signs. Specifically, lyme disease can present with a range of neurologic symptoms including cranial nerve involvement. The presence of an erythematous rash (erythema migrans) following a visit to an endemic area like Orlando raises your suspicion of lyme. Serologic testing for Borrelia burgdorferi antibodies should be performed, and treatment with antibiotics such as doxycycline is warranted if confirmed or given prophylactically.

Cat scratch disease, caused by Bartonella henselae, can lead to Parinaud's oculoglandular syndrome characterized by conjunctival granulomas and preauricular lymphadenopathy. It can also impact cranial nerve function. Serologic testing and azithromycin antibiotic therapy are indicated for confirmed cases.

Although rare due to vaccination, tetanus and botulism can also be considered. Questioning him regarding his past tetanus vaccination is important. Tetanus leads to muscle contracture and although very rare, even cranial nerve involvement is possible which is known as "cephalic tetanus". However, in cephalic tetanus, infection often follows a head injury or the head region and does specifically involve the cranial nerves.

Given his history of diabetes and osteogenesis imperfecta, neuromuscular and metabolic sources need to be considered. Diabetes increases risk for cranial nerve palsies due to microvascular ischemia, with his variable diplopia and severe pain being possible manifestations of ischemic neuropathy. Tight glycemic control and supportive management are essential. Osteogenesis imperfecta predisposes to connective tissue abnormalities and fractures, which could indirectly affect ocular motility. Ensuring adequate bone health and monitoring for any musculoskeletal complications is also important.

In terms of immediate symptomatic management for him, addressing his severe pain and diplopia is your priority. Because of his variable diplopia, prism correction is not an option. Instead, patching will be most effective to help him function while investigating the many possible differentials. Managing his pain is foremost, including non-steroidal anti-inflammatory drugs (NSAIDs) or other pain relief approaches.

Differential Diagnoses and Rationale

- **Intermittent Cranial Nerve Palsy:** Suggested by his variable, transient diplopia and EOM patterns inconsistent with any specific cranial nerve palsy. This indicates transient dysfunction or partial cranial nerve involvement.
- **Lyme Disease:** Considered due to epidemiological factors (recent visit to an endemic area) and initial presentation with an erythematous rash. Lyme can trigger varying diplopia directly through cranial nerve involvement.
- **Tetanus:** Although rare in developed countries due to vaccination, Clostridium tetani should be considered given his recent skin injury. Tetanus can lead to muscle contractures and stiffness, affecting voluntary

muscle movements including extraocular muscle function producing diplopia.

- **Cat Scratch Disease:** Infection by Bartonella henselae can lead to Parinaud's oculoglandular syndrome, which can include ocular manifestations such as conjunctival granuloma and/or local lymphadenopathy. Though less common, it can also affect cranial nerve function.
- **Botulism:** Particularly wound botulism, which results from toxin production in a wound infected with Clostridium botulinum. This toxin can interfere with neurotransmitter release, leading to a descending paralysis that may involve the extraocular muscles.
- **Leptospirosis:** This bacterial infection can trigger a wide range of symptoms depending on the phase of infection, including diplopia if the cranial nerves are affected.
- **Carotid-Cavernous Fistula (CCF):** A possibility given the complexity of his presentation, though typically associated with pronounced proptosis and conjunctival congestion.
- **Cavernous Sinus Thrombosis:** Suspected due to the involvement of multiple cranial nerves and persistent pain, warranting further detailed imaging looking for possible thrombi or other vascular anomalies within the cavernous sinus.

Learning Points

- Recognize the importance of a thorough history and physical examination in individuals presenting with complex ocular symptoms, including diplopia and severe ocular pain.

- Understand the significance of variable ocular misalignment and its implications for underlying etiologies, requiring comprehensive imaging and diagnostic workups.
- Appreciate the role of advanced imaging techniques, including MRI and CT angiography, in identifying and diagnosing underlying causes of variable diplopia and severe ocular pain.

Questions

What key imaging studies are indicated for evaluating variable diplopia and severe ocular pain?

This includes MRI with FIESTA protocol and CT angiography to assess for any vascular anomalies, inflammatory processes, or compressive lesions within the orbit, cavernous sinus, and cranial nerves.

Why is it important to consider lyme disease in his case?

Lyme disease should be considered because it can present with neurologic symptoms, including cranial nerve involvement. This is particularly relevant to individuals with a history of travel or living in endemic areas, with an erythematous rash suggestive of erythema migrans.

How can medical conditions such as diabetes and osteogenesis imperfecta contribute to ocular symptoms?

Diabetes can lead to microvascular changes and ischemic cranial nerve palsies, while osteogenesis imperfecta can predispose to fractures and connective tissue abnormalities which might also influence ocular alignment and neuromuscular control.

What are the differential diagnoses for varying diplopia and severe ocular pain, and how are they distinguished?

Some differential diagnoses with intermittent cranial nerve palsy can include lyme disease, tetanus, cat scratch disease, botulism, leptospirosis, carotid-cavernous fistula, and cavernous sinus thrombosis. They are distinguished by clinical presentation, associated symptoms, imaging findings, and diagnostic tests such as MRI, CT angiography, and serological studies.

A Party Never to Forget

History of Present Illness (HPI)

A 49-year-old man is in your chair after a great Memorial Day weekend, his homemade spicy buffalo wings and various beers from his new brewmeister was a huge hit. Unfortunately, however, a couple days later he developed severe unrelenting nausea and diarrhea. He was diagnosed with viral gastroenteritis at a walk-in urgent care center, but the doctor believed it was likely unrelated to the party since none of the other partiers reported similar issues. After his urgent care visit, the following day he began experiencing transient double vision which progressively worsened, and when looking in the mirror he noticed the right side of his face drooping. In a frenzy he called you right away.

Review of Systems (ROS)

In addition to his gastrointestinal upset, recent diplopia, and facial droop, he describes episodes of vertiginous symptoms and feeling off balance.

Past Medical History (PMH)

His medical history is unremarkable.

Pertinent Family History (FH)

Family history of migraines which are prevalent among his relatives.

Medications and Allergies

He does not take any medications. He has no known allergies to medications, food, or environment.

Ophthalmic Examination

- **Best Corrected Visual Acuity (BCVA):** OD 20/20, OS 20/20.
- **Pupils:** Pupils equal, round, reactive to light and accommodation, no afferent pupillary defect. PERRLA, (-)APD.
- **Extraocular Muscles (EOMs):** Restricted depression in adducted position OD, with oblique diplopia on left gaze
- **Visual Field (VF):** Full OU
- **Intraocular Pressure (IOP):** 15 mmHg OU.
- **Anterior Segment:** Clear cornea, deep and quiet anterior chamber, clear lens OU. No evidence of inflammatory ophthalmopathy OU.
- **Posterior Segment:** Optic nerve, macula, vessels, vitreous, retina unremarkable OU.

- **Optical Coherence Tomography (OCT):** Normal optic nerve and retinal nerve fiber layer (rNFL) OU, macula clear with good foveal contour OU.

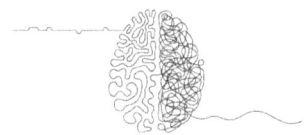

Think Deeper!

His initial presentation suggests a classic viral gastroenteritis, however, his development of neurologic symptoms such as oblique diplopia with facial drooping points you towards something much more ominous.

Given his neurologic presentation, you urgently order an MRI and MRA Brain which proves to be unremarkable without signs of an underlying structural or vascular source. You also order labs including a Complete Blood Count (CBC), Complete Metabolic Panel (CMP/Electrolytes), Erythrocyte Sedimentation Rate (ESR), and C-reactive Protein (CRP). His CBC shows significant leukocytosis indicating a non-specific active inflammatory or infectious process. An elevated sed rate (ESR) was also present, another non-specific marker of generalized inflammation.

In his clinical scenario without a definitive underlying working diagnosis, you must continue to investigate to uncover the neurologic source. Lumbar puncture (LP) will give you a wealth of diagnostic information and is absolutely your next step. LP is a critical diagnostic tool which can provide valuable information about infectious, inflammatory, hemorrhagic, autoimmune, malignant, metabolic, and neurodegenerative conditions affecting the central nervous system. By analyzing the various components of cerebrospinal fluid (CSF), you can more likely narrow down a differential diagnosis, then possibly confirm a working diagnosis to help guide his management.

Several key components are routinely looked for in CSF to provide generalized diagnostic information. Elevated white blood cells (WBCs) indicate infection or inflammatory conditions, while elevated red blood cells (RBCs) suggest hemorrhage. Elevated protein levels are seen in infection, inflammatory conditions, and demyelinating diseases. An elevated protein level without an elevated WBC count is characteristic of Guillain-Barré Syndrome (GBS). Decreased glucose levels are found in bacterial, fungal, and tuberculous infections, whereas viral infections typically show normal glucose levels.

More targeted microbiological methods such as gram staining and cultures help identify bacterial pathogens, and PCR (Polymerase Chain Reaction) identifies viral DNA/RNA such as herpes simplex virus (HSV) and enteroviruses. Antibody and antigen analysis to diagnose specific infections, including the detection of cryptococcal antigen and syphilis antibodies can be performed. Oligoclonal bands and an elevated IgG index are used to diagnose multiple sclerosis and other autoimmune disease. Cytology detects malignant cells in cases of suspected central nervous system (CNS) metastasis.

You consider some of the very high-yield diagnostic information which can be had via LP.

- **Infectious Disease**

CSF analysis in meningitis is essential. Distinguishing between bacterial, viral, fungal, and tuberculous meningitis can be achieved through specific CSF findings. In bacterial meningitis, the CSF typically shows an elevated white blood cell count, predominantly neutrophils, along with elevated protein and decreased glucose levels. Viral meningitis, in contrast, presents with elevated lymphocytes, normal or slightly elevated protein, and normal glucose levels. Fungal and tuberculous meningitis also show elevated lymphocytes and protein but are marked by decreased glucose levels. Encephalitis via a critical infection can manifest with elevated white blood cells and protein in the CSF, with glucose levels that may be normal or decreased. Specific PCR tests can help identify viral causes of encephalitis. For neurosyphilis, a positive venereal disease research laboratory (VDRL) result or fluorescent treponemal antibody absorption (FTA-ABS) in CSF will be diagnostic.

- **Inflammatory Disease**

Lumbar puncture aids in diagnosing inflammatory disease. Multiple sclerosis (MS) is identified by the presence of oligoclonal bands (OCBs) and an elevated immunoglobulin G (IgG) index in CSF. In Guillain-Barré syndrome (GBS), the characteristic finding is albuminocytologic dissociation creating an elevated protein level with a normal or slightly elevated white blood cell count.

- **Subarachnoid Hemorrhage**

In the event of a subarachnoid hemorrhage (SAH), the presence of red blood cells (RBCs) in the CSF that do not clear from the first to the last tube collected is indicative. Additionally, xanthochromia which is a yellow discoloration of the CSF suggests old blood.

- **Autoimmune and Paraneoplastic Disorders**

Autoimmune inflammatory disorders like neuromyelitis optica (NMO) is diagnosed by detecting aquaporin-4 antibodies in the CSF. Paraneoplastic syndromes associated with malignancies can reveal specific antibodies related to the underlying cancer.

- **Malignancies**

In cases of CNS malignancy, the detection of malignant cells in the CSF confirms the diagnosis.

- **Metabolic and Genetic Disorders**

Metabolic and genetic disorders such as leukodystrophies and mitochondrial disease can be identified through specific enzyme deficiencies or genetic markers found in CSF.

- **Neurodegenerative Disorders**

For neurodegenerative conditions like Alzheimer's disease, CSF analysis typically shows decreased levels of amyloid-beta and increased levels of tau protein.

In this gentleman's case, his CSF proved to show markedly increased protein suggesting a polyneuropathic process, commonly associated with an autoimmune response or post-infectious. Given his presentation of oblique diplopia and exam findings suggestive of IVn involvement, as well as him feeling "off balance", Miller-Fisher syndrome (MFS) which is a variant of Guillain-Barre syndrome (GBS) characterized by ophthalmoplegia, ataxia, and areflexia becomes your primary working diagnosis.

This rare condition is often triggered by infection such as Campylobacter jejuni which can be contracted from improperly prepared food. The timing of his gastrointestinal symptoms post-party and his subsequent neurologic manifestations supports your theory. It is a rare acute neuropathy which affects the cranial nerves and sometimes the peripheral nervous system, and is distinguished from other forms of GBS by its unique clinical triad of ophthalmoplegia, ataxia, and areflexia. The pathophysiology of MFS involves molecular mimicry, where the immune system creates antibodies against bacterial components that cross-react with gangliosides, particularly GQ1b in the nervous system. This autoimmune attack results in demyelination and neurologic dysfunction.

Immediate management required is often rapid intervention with intravenous immunoglobulins (IVIG) or plasmapheresis to stop or slow progression and prevent severe complications like respiratory failure. IVIG works by providing a large pool of immunoglobulins which can suppress and neutralize pathogenic autoantibodies and modulate the immune response. Administering IVIG typically involves a dosage of 2g/kg body weight administered over 2-5 days.

Plasmapheresis on the other hand, involves the removal of plasma containing harmful antibodies and replacing it with donor plasma or albumin, thereby reducing the autoimmune attack. The decision to use plasmapheresis involves assessing an individuals overall stability and access to specialized facilities capable of performing this procedure safely.

Management of possible waxing and waning of his signs and symptoms combined with supportive care and rehabilitation is essential for his recovery and long-term management. Supportive care includes maintaining respiratory function, as individuals with MFS are at risk for respiratory muscle weakness. Pulmonary function tests and close monitoring of oxygen saturation are necessary to detect early signs of respiratory compromise.

Rehabilitation involves physical and occupational therapy to address ataxia and muscle weakness. Early intervention with rehabilitative services helps prevent complications such as contractures, muscle atrophy, and day-to-day functional decline. A multidisciplinary team including physiotherapy, occupational therapy, and speech therapy can collaborate to develop an individualized plan focusing on improving his strength, coordination, hopefully leading back to independence.

The prognosis for MFS is generally favorable, often with significant improvement over weeks to months. However, recovery can be variable with some individuals experiencing long-term residual deficits.

Differential Diagnoses and Medical Rationale

- **Miller-Fisher Syndrome (MFS):** Primary consideration given the clinical triad of ophthalmoplegia, ataxia, and areflexia, along with his temporal association of gastrointestinal symptoms suggesting a post-infectious etiology.
- **Guillain-Barre Syndrome (GBS):** Should be considered due to its broader clinical spectrum, but the specific triad of MFS makes it a more likely diagnosis.
- **Botulism:** Considered due to his gastrointestinal symptoms followed by neurologic deficits, but typically presents with descending paralysis and autonomic dysfunction.
- **Myasthenia Gravis:** Can present with ocular symptoms but lacks the ataxia and areflexia characteristics of MFS.
- **Stroke:** Ruled out through neuroimaging, but initially considered due to the acute onset of diplopia and neurologic symptoms.

Learning Points

- Identify the clinical triad of ophthalmoplegia, ataxia, and areflexia in Miller-Fisher syndrome, and understand its association with a post-infectious autoimmune response.
- Understand the mechanisms and indications for IVIG and plasmapheresis in the management of MFS and other autoimmune neuropathies.
- Emphasize the need for early involvement of neurology in diagnosing and managing complex neuropathies to optimize outcomes.

- Recognize the importance of regular follow-up to manage recovery, detect recurrence, and address any residual deficits in patients with MFS.

Questions

What are the key diagnostic investigations for identifying Miller-Fisher syndrome?

Key diagnostics include a complete blood count (CBC) showing leukocytosis, elevated erythrocyte sedimentation rate (ESR), lumbar puncture revealing increased cerebrospinal fluid protein levels, and neuroimaging to rule out structural causes.

Why is early intervention with IVIG or plasmapheresis crucial in managing Miller-Fisher syndrome?

Early intervention with IVIG or plasmapheresis is crucial to reduce the body's autoimmune response, stop progression, and prevent severe complications such as respiratory failure.

What are the differential diagnoses for oblique diplopia and facial drooping, and how are they distinguished?

Differential diagnoses include Guillain-Barre syndrome/Miller-Fisher syndrome, myasthenia gravis, viral meningoencephalitis, and stroke. They are distinguished by clinical presentation, associated symptoms, imaging findings, and diagnostic tests such as CBC, ESR, lumbar puncture, and neuroimaging.

Improving With Time

History of Present Illness (HPI)

A 58-year-old gentleman comes to see you. He tells you over the last several weeks he has been waking up with severe double vision, and also mentions feeling like he hasn't slept because his arms, legs, and body are still tired. It's to the point now where he's actually having difficulty lifting himself out of bed and just wants to lay there for a while. Once he gets moving and "awake", has some coffee, by the time he gets to work all is well for the day.

Review of Systems (ROS)

He's had some occasional night sweats and has lost some weight over the past few months. He has not had any recent fevers or chills. He does have a cough for which he says "because I'm a smoker".

Past Medical History (PMH)

Hypertension and hyperlipidemia for years. Significant smoking history (30 pack-year). He has not seen his family physician in at least 2 years.

Family History (FH)

Father passed away from complications due to prostate cancer. Mother with stroke and now deceased. Both parents with hypertension and hyperlipidemia.

Medications and Allergies

Lisinopril and atorvastatin, with poor compliance. He has no known allergies to medications, foods, or environmental factors.

Ophthalmic Examination

- **Best Corrected Visual Acuity (BCVA):** 20/25 OU.
- **Pupils:** Pupils equal, round, reactive to light and accommodation, no afferent pupillary defect. PERRLA, (-)APD.
- **Extraocular Muscles (EOMs):** Transient paresis and diplopia without a clear pattern.
- **Visual Field (VF):** Full OU.
- **Intraocular Pressure (IOP):** 23 OD, 24 OS.
- **Anterior Segment:** Clear cornea, anterior chamber deep and quiet, early cortical lens changes OU.
- **Posterior Segment:** Optic disc, macula, vessels, vitreous, retina unremarkable OU.
- **Optical Coherence Tomography (OCT):** Normal optic nerve and retinal nerve fiber layer (rNFL) OU, macula clear with good foveal contour OU. No evidence of disc edema OU.

Neurologic Examination

- **Muscle Strength:** 3/5 in both upper and lower extremities.
- **Reflexes:** Normal and symmetrical.
- **Sensation:** Intact throughout.
- **Coordination:** Normal finger-to-nose and heel-to-shin testing.

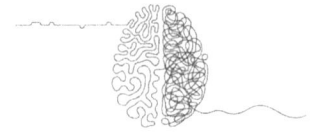

Think Deeper!

Discussion and Management

This gentleman is in your chair with severe diplopia upon awakening. Then intermittent, transient, and variable diplopia found on your exam, which he tells you improves as the day goes on. This is occurring alongside weakness in his extremities but also improving by the end of day.

With his pattern of signs and symptoms, your primary diagnostic thought is the possibility of Lambert-Eaton syndrome, particularly given his long history of smoking and associated weight loss and night sweats.

Lambert-Eaton myasthenic syndrome (LEMS) is a rare autoimmune disorder often linked to small-cell lung carcinoma (SCLC). It involves the production of paraneoplastic antibodies targeting voltage-gated calcium channels (VGCC) present in presynaptic nerve terminals at neuromuscular junctions. These calcium channels are crucial for the release of acetylcholine.

When these calcium channels are under attack by antibodies, the influx of calcium into the nerve terminals is reduced. This diminished calcium influx leads to decreased release of acetylcholine into the synaptic cleft, the neuromuscular junction being the space between nerve and muscle. Consequently, there is insufficient stimulation of muscle fibers resulting in the hallmark symptoms in LEMS of muscle weakness and fatigue.

Symptoms typically begin in the proximal muscles, such as the hips and shoulders, and can improve temporarily with exertion. The characteristic improvement of signs and symptoms throughout the day seems paradoxical, but is due to increased muscle activity physically enhancing calcium influx into presynaptic neurons, improving neuromuscular transmission. This contrasts with myasthenia gravis for which acetylcholine availability becomes reduced, therefore with increased activity acetylcholine is quickly depleted resulting in diminishing muscle function.

The primary diagnostic labs for LEMS involves detecting antibodies against voltage-gated calcium channels (VGCC). These antibodies are found in a significant majority of LEMS patients and are considered a hallmark of the disease. There are two main types of VGCC antibodies that can be identified, P/Q-type and N-type, with P/Q-type VGCC antibodies being more commonly associated with LEMS.

Electromyography (EMG) is a critical tool in the differential diagnosis of LEMS vs myasthenia gravis (MG). EMG will show improving incremental responses to repetitive nerve stimulation in LEMS which will differentiate it from MG. In MG, the EMG will be a diminishing decremental response.

You also consider simple sleep apnea, as it can induce nocturnal hypoxia leading to morning symptoms, but this typically would not account for his pattern and course during the day.

Orthostatic hypotension is your other thought, for which individuals may experience drops in blood pressure during posture changes, especially after awakening and immediately standing. Orthostasis can create transient symptoms but also does not present with his particular pattern.

His unintentional weight loss and night sweats alongside his diplopic pattern makes you suspicious of an underlying malignancy such as SCLC. Therefore, your first and most important step in the diagnostic process is to obtain a high-resolution chest CT or MRI looking for the presence of malignancy, particularly SCLC. If identified and confirmed, staging via PET scan is necessary. Understanding diplopia, MRI brain with and without contrast is also indicated to rule out metastases with cranial nerve involvement, not uncommon in SCLC.

If LEMS is confirmed, treatment may include addressing an underlying malignancy if present. Immunosuppressive therapies such as corticosteroids or azathioprine, and symptomatic treatment with pyridostigmine can be utilized to improve neuromuscular transmission and his symptoms.

Differential Diagnoses and Rationale

- **Paraneoplastic Lambert-Eaton Myasthenic Syndrome (LEMS):** Primary consideration given his history of smoking, intermittent diplopia, morning weakness, weight loss, and night sweats. His improvement of symptoms with activity is characteristic of LEMS.
- **Myasthenia Gravis (MG):** Possible due to the presentation of muscle weakness and diplopia, but

less likely given the improvement with activity as seen in LEMS.

- **Sleep Apnea:** Possible contributor to morning symptoms, though the primary ocular presentation is less typical. Nocturnal hypoxia can lead to morning fatigue and weakness.
- **Orthostatic Hypotension:** Possible contributor to transient symptoms, especially if correlated with changes in posture. However, it does not explain the specific pattern of diplopia and muscle weakness improving with activity.

Learning Points

- Understand the pathophysiology of Lambert-Eaton myasthenic syndrome (LEMS), including its association with small-cell lung carcinoma (SCLC) and the paraneoplastic autoimmune targeting of pre-synaptic calcium channels.
- Recognize the clinical presentation of LEMS, characterized by muscle weakness that improves with activity, and differentiate it from other neuromuscular disorders such as myasthenia gravis.
- Highlight the role of imaging studies, such as high-resolution chest CT or MRI and PET scans, in diagnosing and staging underlying malignancies associated with paraneoplastic syndromes.

Questions

What are key diagnostic investigations for confirming Lambert-Eaton myasthenic syndrome (LEMS)?

Diagnostics for confirming LEMS include high-resolution chest CT or MRI to assess for lung cancer like SCLC, electromyography (EMG) showing improving incremental response to repetitive nerve stimulation, and labs investigating paraneoplastic antibodies targeting neuromuscular pre-synaptic calcium channels.

How can Lambert-Eaton myasthenic syndrome (LEMS) be differentiated from myasthenia gravis (MG)?

LEMS can be differentiated from MG by the characteristic improvement of muscle weakness with activity seen in LEMS, whereas MG typically presents with worsening muscle weakness with activity. EMG findings also differ, with LEMS showing an improving incremental response to repetitive nerve stimulation and MG showing a diminishing decremental response.

Why is it important to assess for underlying malignancies with suspected Lambert-Eaton Myasthenic Syndrome (LEMS)?

It is important to assess for underlying malignancies, particularly small-cell lung carcinoma (SCLC), because LEMS is often a paraneoplastic syndrome associated with malignancy. Identifying and treating the underlying malignancy is crucial for managing LEMS.

Too Twitchy

History of Present Illness (HPI)

A 52-year-old lady is in your chair with concerns about her recurring lower eyelid twitching which has been lingering over the past two months. You automatically ask if it is purely her lid or any other areas of her face or body. She does occasionally have intermittent twitching of her left cheek, and as you're speaking with her you can't help but notice brief involuntary spastic movements of her lid as well as her cheek.

Review of Systems (ROS)

She reports no pain, headaches, or any associated signs or symptoms. However, she does experience occasional bouts of vertiginous type episodes, and has noticed an increase in the frequency and intensity of the spasms. The spasms also seem to occur more when she feels stressed.

Past Medical History (PMH)

Aside from occasional migraines she was diagnosed with years ago, which do not seem coincide with the lid and facial spasms, her medical history is unremarkable. She has no prior neurologic or significant medical illnesses.

Family History (FH)

She has no known family history of neurologic disorders. Both parents are healthy with no significant medical issues.

Medications and Allergies

Occasional acetaminophen or ibuprofen for headaches. She has no known medication or environmental allergies.

Ophthalmic Examination

- **Best Corrected Visual Acuity (BCVA)**: 20/20 OU.

- **Pupils**: Pupils equal, round, reactive to light and accommodation, no afferent pupillary defect. PERRLA, (-)APD.
- **Intraocular Pressure (IOP)**: 15 mmHg OU.
- **Extraocular Muscles (EOMs)**: Full, without diplopia.
- **Visual Field (VF)**: Full OU.
- **Anterior Segment**: Clear cornea, deep and quiet anterior chamber, clear lens OU.
- **Posterior Segment**: Optic nerve, macula, vessels, vitreous, retina unremarkable. No disc edema OU.
- **Optical Coherence Tomography (OCT)**: Normal optic nerve and retinal nerve fiber layer (rNFL) OU, macula clear with good foveal contour OU.

Neurologic Examination

- **Cranial Nerves**: Subtle, involuntary contractions of the orbicularis oculi and zygomatic muscles on the left side, consistent with hemifacial spasm.
- **Facial Nerve**: Increased irritability on the left side.

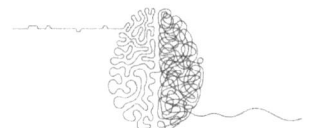

Think Deeper!

Discussion and Management

Her clinical presentation of simultaneous lid and cheek twitching localized to one side of the face, with no other significant neurologic deficits, you strongly suspect a more widespread hemifacial spasm. This is typically triggered by compression of the VIIn, facial nerve, most often at the root exit zone from the brainstem. It is unlike myokymia which generally presents as fine fleeting twitches typically involving only the lids, and also unlike blepharospasm which is bilateral and often associated with other dystonic movements. Hemifacial spasm is instead characterized by unilateral, persistent, and involuntary contractions of the entire facial musculature supplied by the facial nerve.

Given her symptoms, and despite the absence of a pertinent medical or neurologic history, you order an MRI brain with and without contrast with specific focus on the cerebellopontine angle. This imaging will help to visualize the anatomic relationship between the VIIn and adjacent vasculature. In cases of hemifacial spasm, it is not uncommon to find a loop of an arterial vessel compressing the nerve leading to its hyperexcitability. MRI and additional imaging can also rule-out other structural lesions such as masses or vascular malformations which could potentially create a similar clinical scenario.

Your management should be directed towards addressing the root cause of the neuropathy, and if vascular compression is confirmed, microvascular decompression (MVD) offers a viable solution by relieving neuronal compression. This surgical procedure involves repositioning or placing a cushion between the offending vessel and nerve reducing the pressure. The most used material is a small piece of teflon felt. This synthetic material is biocompatible and acts as a cushion to keep the blood vessel separated from the nerve. MVD has a high success rate and can provide permanent relief from hemifacial spasm.

Alternatively, botulinum toxin injections provide symptomatic relief by temporarily paralyzing the overactive facial muscles. Botulinum toxin works by inhibiting the release of acetylcholine at the neuromuscular junction, thereby reducing muscle contractions. This treatment can be beneficial while awaiting more definitive treatment or for individuals who are not candidates for surgery. Botulinum toxin injections typically need to be repeated every three to six months as the effects wear off.

Finally, it is important you address stress as a contributing factor which can exacerbate her symptoms of hemifacial spasm. The relationship between stress and hemifacial spasm is likely multifactorial involving both central and peripheral mechanisms. Stress can increase neurotransmitter levels, enhance blood vessel pulsatility, and affect central nervous system excitability, all of which may contribute to the exacerbation of hemifacial spasm. Stress management techniques, including cognitive-behavioral therapy (CBT), mindfulness, and relaxation exercises, have been shown to help reduce their frequency and severity.

Differential Diagnoses and Medical Rationale

- **Hemifacial Spasm**: Primary diagnosis considered due to her characteristic unilateral lid and facial muscle spasms and typical age of onset. Hemifacial spasm is most often caused by vascular compression of the facial nerve at the root exit zone from the brainstem.

- **Myokymia**: Less likely due to the persistent nature and involvement beyond the her lids. Myokymia typically presents as fine fleeting twitches confined to the lids and is often stress-related or due to fatigue.
- **Blepharospasm**: Unlikely given her unilateral presentation and absence of other dystonic movements. Blepharospasm usually involves both eyes and can be part of a generalized dystonia.
- **Facial Nerve Mass or Other Structural Lesion**: While rare, it remains a differential until imaging definitively rules it out. Masses or other structural lesions can compress the facial nerve leading to similar symptoms.

Learning Points

- Recognize the characteristic presentation of hemifacial spasm, including unilateral, persistent, and involuntary contractions of the lid and facial muscles.
- Understand the importance of MRI, with a focus on the cerebellopontine angle to visualize the anatomic relationship between the facial nerve and adjacent blood vessels and to rule out other structural lesions.
- Emphasize the role of microvascular decompression as a potential definitive treatment for hemifacial spasm caused by vascular compression of the facial nerve.
- Highlight the use of botulinum toxin injections for symptomatic relief, particularly in individuals who are

not candidates for surgery or are awaiting surgical intervention.
- Address the impact of stress on the frequency and severity of hemifacial spasm and the importance of stress management techniques in the overall management plan.

Questions

What imaging modality is recommended for diagnosing hemifacial spasm and why?

MRI and MRA with a focus on the cerebellopontine angle are recommended to visualize the anatomic relationship between the facial nerve and adjacent blood vessels, and to rule out other structural lesions such as masses or vascular malformations.

What is the role of microvascular decompression in the management of hemifacial spasm?

Microvascular decompression (MVD) is a surgical procedure which alleviates pressure on the facial nerve caused by vascular compression, offering a potential solution for hemifacial spasm. MVD involves repositioning or placing a teflon cushion between the offending vessel and nerve.

How do botulinum toxin injections help in managing hemifacial spasm?

Botulinum toxin injections provide symptomatic relief by inducing temporary paresis of overstimulated facial muscles. Botulinum toxin works by inhibiting the release of acetylcholine at the neuromuscular junction reducing muscle contractions.

What are the differential diagnoses for unilateral facial muscle spasms, and how are they distinguished?

Differential diagnoses include hemifacial spasm, myokymia, blepharospasm, and facial nerve mass or structural lesion. Hemifacial spasm is characterized by unilateral, persistent, involuntary contractions of ipsilateral lid and facial muscles, usually due to vascular compression of the facial nerve. Myokymia presents as fine fleeting twitches confined to the lids. Blepharospasm involves bilateral dystonic movements of the lids.

Why is stress management important in the management of hemifacial spasm?

Stress can exacerbate the frequency and severity of hemifacial spasm. Stress management techniques including cognitive-behavioral therapy (CBT), mindfulness, and relaxation exercises can help reduce the impact of stress.

Section 2
Nerve

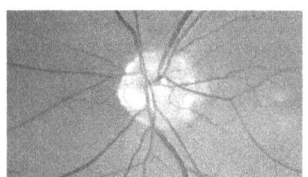

"The study of neurology is the study of the deepest mechanisms of life, consciousness, and human identity."

– Dr. Oliver Sacks

Split Vision

History of Present Illness (HPI)

An 86-year-old lady is in your chair with gastrointestinal symptoms, specifically persistent epigastric discomfort but without nausea or vomiting. She also describes intermittent left flank pain. She underwent an esophagogastroduodenoscopy (EGD) which was inconclusive, however, during the procedure her blood pressure became erratic leading to her being hospitalized overnight. She was discharged and scheduled for a follow-up hepatobiliary iminodiacetic acid (HIDA) scan. 5 days post-discharge, she became diplopic and called you.

Review of Systems (ROS)

She has a history of intermittent dyspepsia and acid reflux, with a recent exacerbation. She denies any changes in bowel habits or urinary symptoms. No recent headaches, syncope, or changes in hearing, although she describes a persistent feeling of fullness in her abdomen. She also feels occasional palpitations.

Past Medical History (PMH)

Intermittent dyspepsia and acid reflux, asthma, hypertension managed with diet and daily walks. She previously had episodes of vertigo which were assessed as benign positional vertigo.

Family History (FH)

Cardiovascular disease, including hypertension and stroke are prevalent in her family.

Medications and Allergies

No regular medications for several years but occasionally uses over-the-counter antacids for her dyspepsia. She does have an allergy to penicillin, no known food or environmental sensitivities.

Ophthalmic Examination

- **Best Corrected Visual Acuity (BCVA):** 20/30 OD, 20/40 OS.
- **Pupils:** Pupils equal, round, reactive to light and accommodation, no afferent pupillary defect. PERRLA, (-)APD.

- **Extraocular Muscles (EOMs):** Restricted abduction OD.
- **Visual Field (VF):** Full OU.
- **Intraocular Pressure (IOP):** 14 mmHg OU.
- **Anterior Segment:** Clear cornea, deep and quiet anterior chamber, pseudophakic OU.
- **Posterior Segment:** Optic nerve with no evidence of disc edema OU. Macular drusen consistent with dry age-related macular degeneration (DAMD) OU. Vessels, vitreous, retina unremarkable OU.
- **Optical Coherence Tomography (OCT):** Normal optic nerve and retinal nerve fiber layer (rNFL) OU. Macular drusen with small RPE detachments OU.

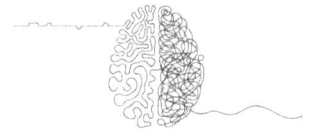

Think Deeper!

Discussion and Management

You must question her acute onset of diplopia following EGD, with your initial thoughts centering around a possible transient vasovagal response to the procedure or an iatrogenic complication. However, her symptoms began 5 days post-procedure, and you then discover a non-transient but persistent isolated right VIn palsy.

The VIn, abducens nerve, is particularly susceptible to ischemic events due to its long intracranial course making it vulnerable to fluctuations in blood pressure and other vascular factors. In elderly individuals, ischemic microvascular infarcts are a common cause of cranial nerve palsies. These events are often related to factors such as hypertension, diabetes, and hyperlipidemia which can compromise small blood vessels supplying the cranial nerves. Despite the 5 day delay, her history of erratic blood pressure during the procedure could have contributed to an ischemic event, for which she is now in your chair with persistent diplopia and a non-improving cranial nerve palsy.

In addition to a potential microvascular infarct, in her case and timeline you must also consider other vascular etiologies. Her unaddressed left flank pain and abdominal "fullness" raises your suspicion with respect to the possibility of an abdominal aortic aneurysm, potentially leading to hemodynamic instability. Therefore, a detailed vascular work-up including abdominal ultrasound and/or CT is warranted. Imaging studies such as a CT angiogram (CTA) of the head and neck are also warranted to further investigate vascular insufficiency as an ischemic source of her VIn palsy.

Cardiology consult is important given the association for cardiac events such as myocardial infarction (MI) to manifest with gastrointestinal and atypical symptoms, especially in females. Specifically the possibility of triggering an ischemic VIn palsy. Therefore, ECG and Echo (echocardiography) is needed looking for cardiac arrhythmia, as well as valvular disease or other structural abnormalities which could lead to embolic phenomena and compromise cerebral perfusion.

Considering her 5 day delay in reporting symptoms, the possibility of an iatrogenic EGD complication with a chronic upper GI bleed creating a severely anemic state, or perforation, and/or septicemia must be considered. CBC with hemoglobin and hematocrit will help tell the story. A chest X-ray, abdominal ultrasound and/or CT is therefore also warranted.

Neuroimaging, specifically MRI with and without contrast of the brain and orbits, should be prioritized to assess for any intracranial pathology such as demyelination, masses, or other structural abnormalities which could impinge on the VI nerve. Given her age and clinical presentation, MRI will provide critical insights into potential neurodegenerative processes or neoplastic conditions which might not be evident on CT imaging alone.

Lumbar puncture may also be considered if you have suspicion of an inflammatory or infectious process. Cerebrospinal fluid (CSF) analysis regarding infection, inflammation, or malignancy can provide valuable diagnostic information, particularly in cases where imaging results are inconclusive.

Provided her diplopia is stable and unchanging, symptomatic management of her VI nerve palsy involves adding prism correction in her glasses. Prism will optically compensate for her ocular misalignment and provide symptomatic relief. Occluding or patching the affected eye is often done initially for at least one month waiting for stability or resolution before prescribing prism. In the case of ischemia or infarction, a 90-day waiting period is widely accepted to learn if there will be resolution. With prism or patching, day to day tasks will be more manageable for her while investigating a final diagnosis and outcome.

Differential Diagnoses and Medical Rationale

- **Microvascular Ischemic Event:** Highly plausible given her age, history of hypertension, erratic blood pressure, and the acute presentation of a VI nerve palsy.
- **Abdominal Aortic Aneurysm:** Hemodynamic instability considered due to her unexplained left flank pain and potential downstream vascular ischemic implications.
- **Cardiac Arrhythmia/Embolic Phenomenon:** Possible given her history of fluctuating blood pressure, pending cardiac consult and evaluation.
- **EGD Complication:** Although rare, complications such as a chromic upper GI bleed, perforation, or septicemia should be ruled out with appropriate labs and imaging.
- **Intracranial Pathology (Masses, Demyelination):** MRI with and without contrast will help identify these potential causes of her VI nerve palsy.

Learning Points

- Understand susceptibility of the VI cranial nerve to ischemic events due to its long intracranial course.
- Evaluate for potential vascular causes such as microvascular ischemia, aneurysms, and cardiac sources of emboli.

- Employ MRI with and without contrast to investigate intracranial pathology and consider additional imaging studies based on your clinical suspicion.
- Utilize prism correction in glasses or temporary occlusion to alleviate diplopia pending the outcome of diagnostic evaluations and a working diagnosis.

Questions

What are key diagnostic investigations for identifying the source of her VIn palsy?

CT head, chest X-ray, ECG, and Echo to identify possible underlying structural, vascular or cardiac issues. CBC looking for blood loss represented by a low hemoglobin and hematocrit.

How can prism help manage diplopia with a VIn palsy and other forms of strabismus?

Prism can help by optically compensating for ocular misalignment eliminating diplopia. This correction may be temporary or permanent depending the etiology, or purely while further diagnostic evaluations and/or treatment are completed.

What are the differential diagnoses for acute diplopia in an elderly patient, and how are they distinguished?

In her scenario, differential diagnoses include a microvascular ischemic event, chronic GI bleed, abdominal aortic aneurysm with hemodynamic instability, cardiac event, and neoplastic causes. They are distinguished by her clinical presentation, associated signs and symptoms, imaging findings, and diagnostics such as appropriate labs, ECG, and Echo.

Droopy Droopy

History of Present Illness (HPI)

A 39-year-old lady is in your chair with the entire left side of her face drooping. She first noticed this while looking in the mirror brushing her teeth the morning before, and then found it difficult to spit. When she looked in the mirror again, her left eye did not want to close. In a panic she immediately called her primary care physician who then sent her to the emergency room under stroke protocol. She's discharged and then calls you confused and fearful, not understanding what is happening to her.

Review of Systems (ROS)

She has difficulty with facial movements on the left side, including trouble blinking or closing her left eye. She tells you that side of her face "doesn't want to smile". She has no weakness or numbness in her arms or legs, slurred speech, or difficulty swallowing. She has not experienced any recent trauma, infection, or rashes. No recent history of headaches, dizziness, or vision change. She has no chest pain, shortness of breath, or palpitations.

Past Medical History (PMH)

She has had episodic migraines but without aura since a teenager. She has no history of hypertension, diabetes, or cardiovascular disease. She suspects seasonal allergies, however, no asthmatic or respiratory issues.

Family History (FH)

Her family history is unremarkable for neurologic disorders or cardiovascular disease. Her father does have a history of mild hypertension.

Medications and Allergies

Over-the-counter ibuprofen and loratadine as needed for her headaches. She has no known allergies to medications, foods, or environmental factors.

Ophthalmic Examination:

- **Best Corrected Visual Acuity (BCVA):** 20/20 OU.
- **Pupils:** Pupils equal, round, reactive to light and accommodation, no afferent pupillary defect. PERRLA, (-)APD.
- **Extraocular Muscles (EOMs):** Full, without diplopia.
- **Visual Field (VF):** Full OU.
- **Intraocular Pressure (IOP):** 21 OD, 20 OS.
- **Anterior Segment:** Cornea clear, deep and quiet anterior chamber, clear lens OU. Lagophthalmos with inferior corneal exposure OS.
- **Posterior Segment:** Optic disc, macula, vessels, vitreous, retina unremarkable OU.
- **Optical Coherence Tomography (OCT):** Normal optic nerve and retinal nerve fiber layer (rNFL) with no evidence of disc edema OU, macula clear with good foveal contour OU.

Neurologic Examination:

- **Cranial Nerves:** Left-sided facial droop with

lagophthalmos OS, and without the ability to raise her left eyebrow. No other cranial nerve deficits evident.

- **Motor and Sensory:** Strength 5/5 in all extremities. Normal sensation throughout.
- **Reflexes:** Normal and symmetric.
- **Coordination:** Normal finger-to-nose and heel-to-shin testing.

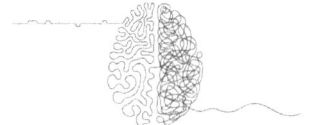

Think Deeper!

Discussion and Management

After an extensive evaluation and imaging in the ER, your patient was found to have Bell's palsy and she comes to see you with classic signs and symptoms. A unilateral left-sided facial droop with an inability to raise her left eyebrow, along with lagophthalmos and corneal exposure.

Despite her recent work-up in the ER clearing her regarding stroke, you immediately recognize the fact stroke is highly unlikely simply by understanding basic anatomic and functional principles of her presentation. Bell's can be distinguished from a central cause like stroke purely due to the fact she has lost the ability to raise her left eyebrow.

Bell's palsy is an acute condition characterized by the sudden onset of a unilateral peripheral facial nerve (VIIn) paralysis or weakness, with no identifiable cause. It typical develops over a period of hours to days. Its precise pathophysiology remains unclear, though it is widely believed to be associated with viral infection. Reactivation of the herpes simplex virus (HSV) or varicella-zoster virus (VZV) within the geniculate ganglion is thought to trigger inflammation and subsequent edema of the facial nerve. This inflammation, coupled with edema, leads neuronal compression within the narrow bony fallopian canal in the temporal bone. The restricted space within the canal exacerbates the compression, potentially resulting in an ischemic event. An autoimmune response has been implicated as well and may contribute to the inflammation and even possible demyelination.

Treatment for Bell's typically involves a combination of medication and physical therapy. Corticosteroids, such as prednisone, are often prescribed to reduce neuronal inflammation and edema. The effectiveness of corticosteroids is maximized when administered early and within 72 hours of symptom onset. In cases where a viral etiology is suspected, antiviral medications such as acyclovir or valacyclovir may be added, although their effectiveness remains debated and are often considered adjunctive rather than primary treatments.

Physical therapy can play an important role in managing recovery. Gentle facial exercises aim to stimulate and strengthen the facial muscles, helping to improve nerve function and prevent muscle atrophy. These exercises involve movements such as smiling, frowning, and raising the eyebrows. Massage therapy can also be beneficial, with gentle massage of the facial muscles helping to reduce stiffness and improve perfusion. In some scenarios, electrical stimulation can be used to enhance muscle activation and nerve function. Additionally, biofeedback techniques, which involve electronic monitoring can teach individuals to control facial muscle movements and improve muscle coordination.

Finally, and very importantly, eye protection including artificial tears and lubricating ointment at bedtime is imperative in the prevention of exposure keratitis. While sleeping, taping the lid closed or wearing a shield creating a "moisture chamber" is also key prophylactic treatment. Exposure keratitis without proper management can progress to dangerous and possibly vision threatening neurotrophic and/or infectious ulceration, scarring, and even potential perforation in extreme cases.

The outcome of Bell's palsy is generally favorable with most individuals recovering fully within three to six months. However, some may experience residual weakness or synkinesis, involuntary facial movements. Early treatment and physical therapy are essential for improving outcomes and reducing the likelihood of long-term complications.

Of course, her initial presentation of a sudden-onset facial droop raised immediate concern for a cerebrovascular event, particularly stroke. Given the suspicion, her primary care physician requested stroke protocol in the ER requiring a full comprehensive work-up, including imaging and labs. While these steps are necessary to rule-out stroke, you are reminded of the high degree of emotional stress, as well as a physical toll, on any individual faced with this potential diagnosis.

In contrast to the anatomic and underlying pathophysiology in Bell's palsy, stroke will instead affect the central VIIn pathway as it travels from the brainstem through the cortex. The forehead and eyebrows are spared due to redundant bilateral VIIn cortical innervation, allowing for preserved brow movement and elevation. Therefore, the inability to raise her eyebrow on the affected side supports a peripheral VIIn palsy over a centrally occurring stroke. This a key distinguishing feature favoring Bell's over stroke, and the differentiation can be made within seconds based on a simple diagnostic check of brow movement.

In retrospect, a more focused neurologic assessment by her PCP and the emergency physician may have eliminated unnecessary extensive diagnostics, as well as saving her from the associated stress, resources, and cost. Although worrisome, a diagnosis of Bell's palsy leads to a much more favorable prognosis and often with full recovery.

Differential Diagnoses and Rationale

- **Bell's Palsy:** The most likely diagnosis given her acute onset of unilateral facial paralysis, lagophthalmos, and lack of eyebrow movement or elevation. This condition is typically idiopathic but often linked to viral infections.
- **Ischemic Stroke:** Although initially suspected, the absence of associated neurologic deficits and her purely peripheral facial nerve involvement points away from stroke. Imaging studies and the ER evaluation cleared her.
- **Lyme Disease:** Can present with facial nerve palsy but typically associated with a history of a tick bit, target lesion, and additional systemic symptoms.

Serologic labs can help rule this out if there is suspicion.

- **Ramsay Hunt Syndrome:** Caused specifically by the varicella-zoster virus (shingles), it presents with a VIIn facial palsy but with a characteristic vesicular rash in the ear canal or on the tympanic membrane. The absence of these lesions makes this diagnosis less likely.
- **Multiple Sclerosis (MS):** While MS can target cranial nerves including the VIIn, it typically presents with other neurologic symptoms and is less likely given her very acute presentation. MRI and further neurologic evaluation can rule this out if necessary.

Learning Points

- Learn to distinguish between Bell's palsy and stroke by noting the involvement of the forehead and eyebrow. In Bell's palsy, there is an inability to raise the eyebrow on the affected side due to purely peripheral facial nerve involvement, whereas stroke will spare the forehead and eyebrows due to redundant VIIn bilateral cortical innervation.
- Understand early treatment with corticosteroids can significantly improve outcomes in Bell's palsy by reducing inflammation and edema facilitating faster recovery of facial nerve function.
- Recognize the priority of reducing risk of permanent vision loss due to exposure keratopathy in lagophthalmos. Preventing permanent corneal scarring or perforation with artificial tears, gels,

ointments, taping, and shields is essential to protect against keratitis and/or its progression.

Questions

What is the primary distinguishing feature of Bell's palsy compared to stroke?

Bell's affects the entire half of the face, including the ipsilateral forehead and eyebrow due to purely peripheral facial nerve involvement. In contrast, stroke spares the forehead and eyebrows due to redundant bilateral cortical innervation.

Why are corticosteroids considered the mainstay of treatment for Bell's palsy?

They help reduce inflammation and edema of the facial nerve, improving the likelihood of a full recovery if initiated promptly.

When should antiviral medications be considered in the treatment of Bell's palsy?

Antivirals may be considered if there is a strong suspicion of a viral etiology, such as herpes simplex or zoster, although their efficacy remains debated.

What supportive measures are important for individuals with Bell's palsy?

Prioritizing eye protection to prevent irreversible keratopathy, scarring, or perforation due to chronic lagophthalmos, using lubricating eye drops during the day, ointments at night, and taping the eyelid shut during sleep.

What are potential differential diagnoses for someone presenting with a sudden unilateral facial droop?

Top differentials include ischemic stroke, Bell's palsy, Ramsay-Hunt syndrome, lyme disease, and demyelinating disease.

Triple Superimposition

History of Present Illness (HPI)

A 45-year-old lady is referred to you by her neurologist due to a longstanding decrease in vision in her left eye. She first noticed a change about two months after undergoing LASIK surgery nearly a decade prior to seeing you. However, over the past several months her vision in that eye has gradually worsened and wonders if her LASIK is "wearing off".

Review of Systems (ROS)

She has experienced prolonged episodes of debilitating muscle aches and pains over the years, which last several days at a time. She also mentions occasional episodes of chest palpitations and instances when she needs to "catch her breath".

Past Medical History (PMH)

She developed polymyositis about two years post-LASIK . About a year ago, she began treatment for a newly diagnosed cardiac arrhythmia and cardiomyopathy, She also has longstanding hypertension which is well controlled.

Family History (FH)

Her mother has a history of rheumatoid arthritis. Both parents have histories of type-2 diabetes, hypertension, and hyperlipidemia.

Medications and Allergies

Cellcept for polymyositis and lifetime anti-coagulation, Eliquis and metoprolol for her arrhythmia. She has no known allergies to medication or environment.

Ophthalmic Examination

- **Best Corrected Visual Acuity (BCVA):** 20/20 OD, 20/40- OS.
- **Pupils:** Pupils equal, round, reactive to light and accommodation (PERRLA); presence of a mild relative afferent pupillary defect, (+)APD OS.
- **Extraocular Muscles (EOMs):** Full, without diplopia.
- **Visual Field (VF):** Full OD. General mild constriction OS.
- **Intraocular Pressure (IOP):** 14 mmHg OD, 13 mmHg OS.
- **Anterior Segment:** Clear cornea, deep and quiet anterior chamber, clear lens OU.
- **Posterior Segment:** Optic nerve unremarkable OD, Optic nerve cupping and pallor OS. Macula, vessels, vitreous, retina unremarkable OU.
- **Optical Coherence Tomography (OCT):** OCT normal optic nerve OD, good foveal contour OU. Retinal nerve fiber layer (rNFL) thinning with advanced cupping and decreased rim volume OS.

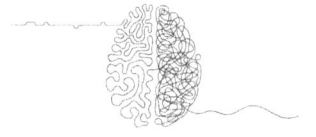

Think Deeper!

Discussion and Management

Your patient presents with a seemingly straightforward history; however, her complex medical background adds significant layers to her differential diagnoses and management. Her OCT imaging shows a compromised rNFL and increased cupping with decreased rim volume in the left eye, suggesting several potential differential diagnoses including previous optic neuritis, superimposed non-arteritic vs arteritic ischemic optic neuropathy (NAION vs AION), and possibly superimposed normal-tension glaucoma (NTG).

Given her history of polymyositis, you know there is a real possibility her vision loss may be related to an autoimmune-mediated process, specifically demyelinating in nature. MRI of the brain and orbits is therefore essential, which you ordered, revealing subtle changes in white matter possibly consistent with demyelination. Considering her cardiac history and recent onset of arrhythmia, her differential must also include non-arteritic chronic ischemia from circulatory insufficiency and/or micro-embolic events.

The progressive nature of her symptoms suggests to you superimposed normal-tension glaucoma over time, due to an already compromised optic nerve. This contrasts with ischemic events, as well as recurrent events such as optic neuritis, which typically present with acute or compounding vision loss rather than a gradual decline. Glaucomatous optic neuropathy, on top of possibly pre-existing inflammatory and/or ischemic optic neuropathy leading to progressive vision loss, is consistent with her clinical picture.

Integrating her care involves bringing on board general neurology for further evaluation in terms of managing this potential overlap of autoimmune dysregulation, cardiovascular instability, and her glaucomatous optic neuropathy. You also obtain visual evoked potentials (VEP), which indeed confirms a delay in the affected eye supporting a true optic neuropathy.

Her clinical course underscores the necessity of integrating these additional diagnostic investigations to fully address the multifaceted nature of her presentation. MRI and MRA are critical to assess for demyelinating brain and/or cervical spine lesions or vascular anomalies. A carotid ultrasound is necessary to evaluate for vascular stenosis or plaque formation which could compromise cerebral or optic nerve perfusion. ECG and Echo need to be revisited to determine her status with regard to cardiomyopathy. Labs including general inflammatory markers such as ANA, ESR, CRP, as well as a complete blood panel, CBC and CMP, are essential to help target possible infectious and/or additional inflammatory processes. Lipid panel is necessary. A COAG, coagulopathy panel is important. Lyme as well as COVID or COVID vaccine can also be a trigger in inflammatory ophthalmopathy. Lyme titers can be ordered. Finally, in addition to measuring opening CSF pressure, LP/lumbar puncture looking for "oligoclonal banding" is the gold standard in ruling-in or ruling-out active demyelination.

Your management strategies must be comprehensive, targeting not only her ocular findings, but as always the true source. Immunomodulatory therapy will likely be indicated if her findings supports a diagnosis of demyelination. Protecting the integrity of the optic nerve is of course key, whether it be via traditional IOP lowering, or in her case with normal IOP, novel neuroprotection. This includes topical treatment such as latanoprostene bunod, which may target both by lowering intraocular pressure as well as potentially enhancing ocular perfusion to the posterior pole and optic nerve. Latanoprostene bunod's additional nitric oxide mechanism of action supports potential increased perfusion.

Her clinical scenario nicely illustrates the integration of ophthalmic medicine, general medicine, and neurology, emphasizing the importance of a thorough and methodical approach to diagnosis and management.

She is also a reminder to not permit patients to sway you by telling you what they think is their diagnosis. For example, in this case assuming her problem is LASIK/cornea related will lead you far away down the wrong path.

Differential Diagnoses and Medical Rationale

- **Optic Neuritis:** Characterized by acute inflammation of the optic nerve, which can lead to sudden vision loss, pain (or no pain) with eye movement, as well as a characteristic afferent pupillary defect. Red desaturation is also a tell-tell symptom of optic neuropathy. Her history of polymyositis, an autoimmune condition, raises the likelihood of optic neuritis which is also often autoimmune-mediated and related to demyelinating disease such as multiple sclerosis.

- **Ischemic Optic Neuropathy:** Both arteritic (AION) and non-arteritic (NAION) forms are possible diagnoses. Her presentation and cardiovascular history point towards a non-arteritic component. NAION is associated with underlying vascular disease which can lead to sudden vision loss without pain, often seen in individuals like her with cardiac issues, hypertension, diabetes, and/or hyperlipidemia.

- **Normal Tension Glaucoma (NTG):** Progressive optic neuropathy with a characteristic cupping pattern and thinning of the rNFL, confirmed with OCT, is likely linked to her underlying vascular dysregulation. This form of glaucoma occurs despite intraocular pressure being within normal range (<21mmHg), often associated with vascular compromise affecting optic nerve perfusion. The progressive nature of her symptoms supports NTG over time due to an already compromised optic nerve. This contrasts with recurrent optic neuritis and/or ischemic events, which will be episodic and acute in nature.

- **Optic Neuritis + NAION + NTG:** A triple superimposition.

- **Post-LASIK Ectasia:** A consideration due to the time of initial symptoms post-LASIK, though less likely given her new onset of symptoms and clinical findings. Corneal ectasia is a rare but serious complication following LASIK surgery, characterized by progressive thinning and bulging of the cornea, leading to visual disturbances.

Learning Points

- Optic neuritis is characterized by acute inflammation of the optic nerve, leading to symptoms such as sudden decreased vision, red desaturation, pain with or without eye movement, and an afferent pupillary defect. Given her autoimmune background and MRI findings, this remains a concern.
- Ischemic optic neuropathy, both arteritic and non-arteritic forms should be considered, particularly with her hypertensive and cardiac history.
- Normal tension glaucoma (NTG) can create progressive optic neuropathy with a characteristic cupping pattern representing neuro-retinal rim thinning, often linked to systemic vascular dysregulation. The progressive nature of her symptoms leans towards NTG over time due to an already compromised optic nerve.
- Post-LASIK ectasia, although less likely in her case, should be considered in individuals with a history of LASIK surgery and subsequent visual disturbances.

Questions

What are hallmark signs of optic neuritis on physical examination?

Hallmark signs include sudden reduced visual acuity with or without pain, red desaturation, relative afferent pupillary defect (RAPD), and possible optic disc edema and/or pallor on retinal examination depending on severity and timing.

Why is her family history significant?

Her family history is significant because autoimmune disease, such as rheumatoid arthritis in her mother, can suggest a predisposition to autoimmune conditions including optic neuritis, MS, and others.

What is the role of MRI in her evaluation?

MRI of the brain and orbits with contrast is crucial to identify signs of inflammatory demyelinating activity, or structural abnormalities affecting her optic nerve and/or visual pathway, which can be indicative of conditions like optic neuritis and multiple sclerosis.

What are key features of normal-tension glaucoma (NTG)?

Key features of NTG include progressive glaucomatous optic neuropathy with characteristic cupping, rNFL thinning on OCT, visual field loss, but with normal intraocular pressure (<21mmHg). It is often associated with underlying cardiovascular factors affecting optic nerve perfusion.

Toddler "Headbutt"

History of Present Illness (HPI)

A 24-year-old young lady comes to your office early in the morning outside of regular hours in a state of panic. Her vision suddenly blurred out in her left eye after her toddler accidentally "head-butted" her the previous evening. It was a hard direct hit, and she is still blurred with pain around that eye.

Review of Systems (ROS)

You ask her about the exact type of pain she is experiencing, whether it's a scratchy surface foreign body sensation, an ache, or pressure type pain. She has no diplopia, visual field deficit, loss of vision, flashes or floaters in that eye. No paresthesia, limb weakness, or balance issues. She has never experienced anything like this before. It is a constant achy pain around her eye that seems worse when she looks side to the side, as well as blurred vision.

Past Medical History (PMH)

She has a generally unremarkable medical history with no prior significant illnesses. She had a full-term, uncomplicated pregnancy and is a mom to her 18-month-old daughter.

Family History (FH)

Her mother had been diagnosed with systemic lupus erythematosus (SLE), and she remembers her maternal aunt having unusual medical issues requiring frequent doctor visits.

Medications and Allergies

She occasionally uses Tylenol for headaches. She has no known allergies to medications or environmental issues.

Ophthalmic Examination

- **Best Corrected Visual Acuity (BCVA):** 20/20 OD; 20/200 OS.
- **Red Desaturation:** Marked red desaturation OS vs OD.
- **Pupils:** Pupils equal, round, reactive to light and accommodation (PERRLA); presence of relative afferent pupillary defect. (+)RAPD OS.
- **Extraocular Muscles (EOMs):** Full, without diplopia. (+) Pain on movement OS.
- **Visual Field (VF):** Full OD. Generalized constriction OS.
- **Intraocular Pressure (IOP):** 16 mmHg OD; 17 mmHg OS.
- **Anterior Segment:** Clear cornea, deep and quiet anterior chamber, clear lens OU. No sign of trauma such as uveitis or hyphema OU.
- **Posterior Segment:** Optic nerve unremarkable OD, disc edema OS. Macula, vessels, vitreous, retina without evidence of traumatic injury such as holes, tears, hemorrhages, detachment, or edema (Berlins edema) OU.
- **Optical Coherence Tomography (OCT):** OD unremarkable. OS reveals thinning of the retinal nerve fiber layer (rNFL) as well as disc edema. Macula with good foveal contour without edema OU.

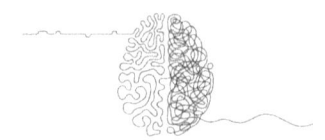

Think Deeper!

Discussion and Management

Her sudden drop in vision with pain on movement, particularly in the presence of an relative afferent pupillary defect (RAPD), disc edema, and retinal nerve fiber layer (rNFL) thinning on OCT, tells you to put your neuro-ophthalmic hat on. Given her family history of autoimmunity and this type of acute presentation, your top differential first leans heavily towards retro-bulbar optic neuritis vs a severe enough injury to produce a traumatic optic neuropathy. Possibly linked to a broader autoimmune or demyelinating process, you consider her demographic for which demyelinating disease such as multiple sclerosis (MS) is often first found.

Optic neuritis is characterized by inflammation of the optic nerve, usually presenting with acute vision loss, red desaturation, without pain or with pain (retro-bulbar) upon eye movement, and a RAPD. Its association with demyelinating disease like MS makes this scenario particularly concerning, as it could signify its first manifestation for her. Her mother's history of SLE further raises your suspicion of an autoimmune etiology.

Your next step involves urgent neuroimaging, specifically MRI of the brain and orbits with contrast, looking for retro-bulbar inflammation along the visual pathway as well as potential evidence of demyelinating lesions. MRI is the gold standard for diagnosing optic neuritis and can reveal areas of demyelination consistent with MS or other demyelinating disease. If imaging shows new or enhancing lesions consistent with demyelination, additional autoimmune and inflammatory markers in the blood including non-specific antinuclear antibody (ANA), and more specific aquaporin-4 antibodies, must also be investigated with respect to neuromyelitis optica spectrum disorder (NMOSD) and related conditions. NMOSD is an additional entity which can present with similar symptoms but requires different management strategies.

Inflammation in optic neuritis is driven by an autoimmune response and involves the degradation of its protective myelin sheath. In the case of MS which frequently accompanies optic neuritis, the immunopathology involves activation of T-cells and other immune mediators which cross the blood-brain barrier leading to areas of cortical demyelination and potentially targeting the optic nerve.

In addition to the degradation of the myelin sheath, there is often direct axonal injury. This axonal target is a critical factor in determining the extent and permanence of vision loss. While myelin can regenerate to some extent, axonal injury can lead to more permanent deficits.

Another key player in this process is microglia, the resident immune cells of the central nervous system. In response to inflammation, microglia become activated and release cytokines and other inflammatory mediators which exacerbate tissue damage to both the myelin sheath and axons.

The integrity of the blood-brain barrier may also be compromised, permitting additional infiltration into the central nervous system only exacerbating the inflammatory process. This further amplifies the autoimmune attack on the optic nerve.

Persistent inflammation and repeated episodes of optic neuritis can lead to chronic neurodegenerative changes. Over time, this can result in permanent rNFL thinning and defects with loss of retinal ganglion cells which are critical for transmitting visual information. Additionally, the inflammatory process generates oxidative stress which contributes to further neuronal damage. Reactive oxygen species produced can damage additional cellular components, also exacerbating the optic neuropathy.

The pathophysiology of optic neuritis is therefore a complex interplay of immune-mediated demyelination, axonal damage, microglial activation, disruption of the blood-brain barrier, and oxidative stress. These mechanisms collectively impair transmission of visual information from the eye to the brain, resulting in the clinical manifestations of optic neuritis. These processes are also crucial targets in therapies which can mitigate damage and improve visual outcomes.

In terms of your management with MRI confirmed retrobulbar optic neuritis, standard protocol begins with high-dose intravenous corticosteroids reducing the targeted immune response, hopefully preserving nerve function. Treatment typically is methylprednisolone 1 gram intravenously daily for 3-5 days, followed by an oral taper. This can accelerate visual recovery and reduce the severity of the episode; however, it does not change the long-term prognosis or risk of future MS complications. Continuous management and follow-up are essential to assess response to treatment and adjust as necessary based on the evolving clinical picture. This includes repeat acuity, visual field, and optic nerve OCT over time to manage any changes, and in her case hopefully resolution.

Understanding the dynamics and unpredictability in immunopathology, additional labs including rheumatoid factor (RF), anti-cyclic citrullinated peptide (anti-CCP), and anti-Smith antibodies, should be considered to comprehensively investigate co-existing processes. The presence of these findings can indicate more widespread disease requiring targeted medical therapy. If the diagnosis of MS or NMOSD is confirmed, longer term disease modifying therapies may need to be started.

It is important you are empathetic and understanding regarding the implications of her potential diagnosis. Discussing possible long-term outcomes, including confirmation or risk of developing clinically significant MS will help prepare her for ongoing lifetime management. Supportive care, sometimes including psychological support may be necessary to address any anxiety and ensure she feels supported.

Differential Diagnoses and Medical Rationale

- **Optic Neuritis:** Primary consideration given her demographic as a younger female, with clinical findings and family history suggesting an autoimmune source. Her acute drop in vision, presence of a RAPD, red desaturation, and optic disc edema and/or pallor are classic signs and symptoms.
- **Traumatic Optic Neuropathy:** Although less likely, physical trauma from her toddler could theoretically precipitate an acute traumatic optic neuropathy.
- **Neurologic Conditions:** Given the sudden onset, and/or if a specific neurologic visual field defect is present, differentials which could create similar

presentations such as an acute ischemic optic neuropathy or stroke can be considered and ruled-out through imaging and clinical correlation. An acute ischemic event could occur, but less likely in her case as an otherwise young healthy individual.

Learning Points

- Understand her clinical presentation of optic neuritis which includes acute vision loss, red desaturation, pain upon eye movement, presence of a relative afferent pupillary defect (RAPD), and disc edema. Pain with eye movement is consistent with retrobulbar activity.
- Appreciate the significance of her family history of autoimmune disease, systemic lupus erythematosus (SLE), which can predispose her to autoimmune conditions like optic neuritis and multiple sclerosis (MS).
- Know the importance of MRI brain and orbits with contrast to diagnose optic neuritis and assess for signs of demyelination and/or structural abnormalities.
- Recognize the role of high-dose intravenous corticosteroids in the acute management of optic neuritis to reduce the immunopathologic response and accelerate visual recovery. Typical treatment is methylprednisolone 1 gram intravenously daily for 3-5 days, followed by an oral taper.

Questions

What are hallmark signs and symptoms of optic neuritis on her physical examination?

Hallmark signs include acute reduction in visual acuity, red desaturation, relative afferent pupillary defect (RAPD), with possible optic disc edema and/or pallor. This can occur with or without pain. If pain, it is likely retrobulbar for which the optic nerve may appear normal on exam.

Why is family history significant in her case?

Her family history is significant because autoimmune disease, such as systemic lupus erythematosus (SLE) in her mother, can suggest a predisposition to autoimmunity. This includes optic neuritis, MS, and other demyelinating disease.

What is the role of MRI in her work-up?

MRI of the brain and orbits with contrast is crucial to identify signs of inflammatory lesions or structural abnormalities affecting her optic nerve and/or visual pathways, indicative of conditions like optic neuritis or multiple sclerosis.

Catching A Wave

History of Present Illness (HPI)

Your first patient of the morning is a 44-year-old gentleman who comes to see you with new onset blurred and distorted vision in his right eye, which started the evening before. He has no associated pain and tells you his vision is no different than when he first noticed it, except when he first woke up straight lines now appear wavy. He was referred to you by your nearby local urgent care.

Review of Systems (ROS)

He has been experiencing occasional headaches and tells you about losing weight over the past few months. He has not changed his diet and does not exercise. He mentions some mild dizziness and occasional palpitations, which is new. No recent fevers, chills, or night sweats.

Past Medical History (PMH)

He has a history of hypertension with questionable control. He was recently evaluated for persistent fatigue, but no definitive diagnosis was made.

Family History (FH)

Father with hypertension, type-2 diabetes, hyperlipidemia, and recent stroke. Mother has age-related macular degeneration (ARMD) but no medical issues.

Medications and Allergies

No medications, non-compliant with previous medication for hypertension. No known allergies to medications, foods, or environmental factors.

Ophthalmic Examination:

- **Best Corrected Visual Acuity (BCVA):** 20/25 OD, 20/20 OS
- **Pupils:** Pupils equal, round, reactive to light and accommodation, no afferent pupillary defect. PERRLA, (-)APD.

- **Extraocular Muscles (EOMs):** Full, no diplopia.
- **Visual Field (VF):** Full OU.
- **Intraocular Pressure (IOP):** 17 OD, 18 OS.
- **Anterior Segment:** Clear cornea, deep and quiet anterior chamber, clear lens OU.
- **Posterior Segment:** Optic nerve, vessels, vitreous, retina unremarkable OU. Mild macular changes with obscured foveal reflex and hyper-reflectance OD. Macula clear OS.
- **Optical Coherence Tomography (OCT):** Normal optic nerve and retinal nerve fiber layer (rNFL) OU. Mild thickening and wrinkling of the inner macula OD. No evidence of disc edema OU.

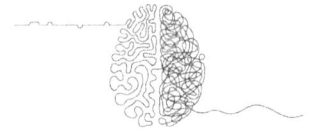

Think Deeper!

Discussion and Management

His OCT findings suggest an epiretinal membrane (ERM), however, you know this typically creates a more gradual onset of decreasing vision or metamorphopsia rather than sudden symptoms. Therefore, you cannot comfortably assume ERM is the etiologic source for him.

With such an acute change in vision along with some form of obscuration only in his right eye, you must first rule-out an ischemic event, despite the obvious ERM on exam. Understanding his non-compliance with treatment for hypertension, knowing to assume nothing, you decide to send him to the ER under stroke protocol.

In the ER he was admitted, ECG performed and placed on a monitor, echocardiogram, carotid duplex, labs including coagulation studies, as well as CT head was completed. A source of a possible acute ischemic event, such as an ischemic optic neuropathy, was not found. However, his blood pressure was mildly elevated for which he was placed back on medication.

With an ischemic source ruled-out, your focus shifts to other potential diagnoses. Given his weight loss, headaches, and mild vertiginous symptoms, your investigations are not yet complete. You order a follow-up MRI brain with and without contrast looking for a more neurologic basis, including demyelination or space-occupying mass.

Regarding optic neuritis and/or demyelinating disease, MRI will help you better assess vs CT. A comprehensive metabolic panel (CMP), complete blood count (CBC), thyroid panel, ANA, ESR, CRP needs to be reviewed or ordered to investigate many other conditions possibly contributing to his clinical picture. Additionally, lyme disease is a consideration and lyme IGG/IGM titers should be obtained.

With his current VA in that eye at 20/25, adopting a watchful waiting approach with close management in terms of vision changes is reasonable. If you suspect demyelination or multiple sclerosis on MRI, oral steroids should be avoided due to the risk of recurrence. However, if there is progression to significant vision loss (worse than 20/40), and a new diagnosis of demyelination within 30 days of his initial symptoms, intravenous corticosteroid treatment is standard protocol.

If lyme disease or a viral etiology is suspected or confirmed creating an optic neuritis, it can be supported by lymphocytosis such as in EBV, HZV, and others. In the case of lyme, doxycycline is the treatment of choice.

Differential Diagnoses and Rationale

- **Epiretinal Membrane (ERM):** His OCT findings and visual symptoms suggest ERM, however, the sudden onset of symptoms point away from this diagnosis as the primary cause.
- **Optic Neuritis:** Given his acute drop in vision despite a normal appearing optic nerve, and despite no pain common with acute retrobulbar optic neuritis. It is still a possibility.
- **Multiple Sclerosis (MS):** If demyelinating lesions are found on MRI, this will point towards MS as the underlying cause triggering an optic neuritis.
- **Non-Arteritic Anterior Ischemic Optic Neuropathy (NAION):** Initially considered due to the acute onset but ruled-out by a negative workup on hospital admission.
- **Lyme Optic Neuritis:** Possible given his symptomatology and if in an endemic area. IGM/IGG lyme titers are necessary.
- **Viral Optic Neuritis:** EBV, HZV, and others can be the source of optic neuritis; CBC with differential looking for lymphocytosis will aid in diagnosis.
- **Idiopathic:** If in the absence of definitive findings.

Learning Points

- Recognize the clinical presentation of an epiretinal membrane, which includes symptoms like blurred and distorted vision with straight lines being seen as wavy (metamorphopsia). Early identification on retinal examination, and OCT for accurate diagnosis and timely intervention.
- Understand the importance of differentiating between acute-onset visual changes and those due to chronic conditions. While ERM typically causes gradual changes, the sudden onset of symptoms necessitates ruling out acute causes such as an ischemic or inflammatory event.
- Recognize the need for a pertinent and complete medical evaluation with acute visual disturbances, especially in individuals with risk factors like hypertension, diabetes, hyperlipidemia, unexplained weight loss, malignancies, and others.
- Appreciate the role of imaging techniques such as MRI of the brain and orbits, as well as detailed labs including CBC, CMP, thyroid function, and others. These investigations help rule-out or support neurologic, vascular, and other systemic causes of visual disturbances.

Questions

What are key features of an epiretinal membrane (ERM) on OCT?

This includes mild thickening and wrinkling of the macular

region, which can create visual distortion (metamorphopsia) and decreased visual acuity.

Why is it important to consider underlying medical conditions in his case?

His symptoms, such as unexplained weight loss, headaches, and mild dizziness strongly indicate a systemic source contributing to his visual disturbances.

What diagnostic investigations are pursued for evaluating potential optic neuritis?

This includes MRI of the brain and orbits with and without contrast, visual evoked potentials (VEP) can support the diagnosis of optic neuritis and other optic neuropathies.

How can lyme disease trigger optic neuritis?

Neurologic manifestations such as optic neuritis are possible in lyme, and should be considered especially in endemic areas.

What is the significance of investigating or ruling-out non-arteritic anterior ischemic optic neuropathy (NAION) in his case?

It is significant because it helps narrow down potential sources of his symptoms, and directs the diagnostic focus towards other etiologies such as demyelinating disease.

No Left Turns

History of Present Illness (HPI)

A 60-year-old lady comes to see you noticing a change in vision in her left eye, she describes it as being "down on my left". Two weeks prior she underwent a lumbar laminectomy and believes the following day is when it first started. She's unsure how to explain it and whether it's blurred or dimmed. Her lumbar region at the surgical site is sill a bit tender, however, her spine surgeon was happy with the procedure and result.

Review of Systems (ROS)

She has no additional symptoms, such as headache, scalp tenderness, jaw claudication, or other suspected neurologic deficits. No fever, weight loss, or night sweats. She has no vertiginous symptoms or balance issues. Her lumbar spinal region is tender post laminectomy.

Past Medical History (PMH)

She has chronic lumbar spinal stenosis and degenerative disc disease, which led to significant lower back pain and radiculopathy. Increasing difficulty walking and doing things at home ultimately led to recent lumbar laminectomy. She also has a history of hypertension, hyperlipidemia, and type-2 diabetes which have been successfully managed with medication.

Family History (FH)

Mother and father with hypertension. Father with type-2 diabetes, hyperlipidemia, and previous stroke.

Medications and Allergies

Metformin 500 mg twice daily, lisinopril 20 mg, atorvastatin 40 mg, and aspirin 81 mg daily. She has no known allergies to medications, foods, or environmental factors.

Ophthalmic Examination

- **Best Corrected Visual Acuity (BCVA):** 20/20 OD, 20/200 OS.
- **Pupils:** Relative afferent pupillary defect present in the left eye. PERRLA, (+)APD OS.
- **Extraocular Muscles (EOMs):** Full, no diplopia.
- **Visual Field (VF):** Full OD. Inferior altitudinal defect OS.
- **Intraocular Pressure (IOP):** 15 OD, 12 OS.
- **Anterior Segment:** Clear cornea, deep and quiet anterior chamber, early nuclear lens changes OU.
- **Posterior Segment:** Hypoplastic "disc-at-risk", macula, vessels, vitreous, retina, unremarkable OD. Disc edema and pallor OS. Macula, vessels, vitreous, retina clear OS. No evidence of diabetic or hypertensive retinopathy OU.
- **Optical Coherence Tomography (OCT):** rNFL thinning with defect OD. Normal optic nerve and retinal nerve fiber layer (rNFL) OS, macula clear with good foveal contour OU.

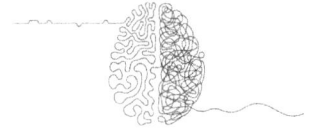

Think Deeper!

Discussion and Management

You have a lady in your chair with a complex presentation, and what she believes as left-sided vision loss following her lumbar laminectomy, raising the possibility of several differential diagnoses. However, on exam, your findings are most consistent with a classic ischemic optic neuropathy with reduced VA, afferent pupillary defect, an inferior altitudinal visual field defect, as well as optic disc edema and pallor.

Non-arteritic anterior ischemic optic neuropathy (NAION) versus a posterior ischemic optic neuropathy (PION) are your top differentials. NAION typically presents with sudden painless vision loss, often upon awakening, and is associated with underlying risk factors such as hypertension, diabetes, and hyperlipidemia, all of which she has a history of. In addition, recent surgery, particularly spinal or cardiac surgery can also precipitate an ischemic event related to potential perioperative hypotension and/or blood loss. NAION following spinal surgery is rare but documented. A disruption in optic nerve perfusion, particularly affecting the anterior portion via the short posterior ciliary arteries can trigger this occurrence.

Predisposing anatomical factors also play a role. A significant risk factor is what is known as "disc-at-risk," which refers to an anatomically crowded optic nerve characterized by a non-existent or small cup-to-disc ratio. Even minor ischemic variations or events can result in significant neuropathy due to limited physical space and natural "compression" within the optic nerve.

Microvascular compromise is a critical aspect of NAION's pathophysiology. Vascular endothelial dysfunction leads to a disruption of the blood-retinal barrier, resulting in localized capillary dropout and peripapillary infarction. The optic nerve contains watershed zones, areas where blood supply from different arterial branches overlap, making these regions particularly susceptible to ischemic injury.

With respect to the optic nerve, an ischemic "event" means axonal injury of optic nerve fibers leading to localized infarction. This in turn triggers a cascade of intracellular metabolic disturbances, including ATP depletion, increased intracellular calcium, and activation of proteolytic enzymes, which contribute to cellular apoptosis and necrosis (cell death) within the optic nerve.

Optic disc edema, a hallmark of acute NAION, results from subsequent axoplasmic flow stasis inducing axonal edema. This further impedes blood flow exacerbating the ischemic injury. Optic disc edema can be quite obvious on exam.

Secondary injury mechanisms involve inflammatory and oxidative stress responses. Ischemia-reperfusion injury can occur when blood flow is transiently restored, intensifying the damage through the production of reactive oxygen species (ROS) and the release of pro-inflammatory cytokines. These processes lead to further neuronal injury perpetuating the cycle of damage.

The possibility of visual recovery in NAION depends on the degree of initial ischemic damage and efficiency of subsequent natural axonal repair mechanisms. Unfortunately, many individuals are left with permanent visual deficits. Moreover, there is a notable risk of NAION affecting the fellow eye, especially in individuals with underlying vascular risk factors and an anatomic "disc-at-risk".

At her age, you consider the possibility of giant cell arteritis (GCA) or temporal arteritis, especially presenting with sudden vision loss. GCA is a vasculitis of medium and large arteries which can lead to an "arteritic" form of ischemic optic neuropathy (AION). Symptoms such as headache, scalp tenderness, jaw claudication, and labs revealing elevated erythrocyte sedimentation rate (ESR) or C-reactive protein (CRP) will support this diagnosis. However, the absence of these symptoms and a normal ESR would make this diagnosis less likely. Temporal artery biopsy remains the gold standard for diagnosing temporal arteritis, if your findings and clinical suspicion warrants it.

Although less common, you also consider a posterior ischemic optic neuropathy (PION). This can occur after significant blood loss and hypotension which was possible during her laminectomy. This can create a retrobulbar ischemic event, posterior to the globe. MRI and MRV of the brain and orbits are necessary for the diagnosis of PION, being it presents without visible optic disc changes initially making imaging studies key in the differential.

Your management of probable NAION primarily focuses on controlling underlying cardiovascular and medical conditions to prevent further episodes. In her case, this includes optimizing blood pressure, glucose, and lipid levels. Additionally, discussing with her perioperative blood pressure management in future surgeries is important to mitigate risks. For PION, immediate management includes stabilizing underlying conditions and addressing reversible causes of hypotension or ischemia due to blood loss.

Differential Diagnoses and Rationale

- **Non-Arteritic Anterior Ischemic Optic Neuropathy (NAION):** The most likely diagnosis given her recent lumbar laminectomy, which could lead to perioperative hypotension and subsequent optic nerve ischemia. The presence of vascular risk factors such as hypertension, diabetes, and hyperlipidemia further support this diagnosis, as well as her anatomical hypoplastic optic nerve in each eye.
- **Posterior Ischemic Optic Neuropathy (PION):** Considered due to the nature of her recent surgery, potential perioperative hypotension, combined with significant blood loss if this occurred. MRI and MRV is necessary to confirm.
- **Temporal Arteritis/Giant Cell Arteritis (GCA):** Less likely in the absence of symptoms such as headache, scalp tenderness, jaw claudication, and elevated ESR/CRP but should still be considered in your differential. Temporal artery biopsy will be necessary for definitive diagnosis if labs results and your clinical findings support it.
- **Optic Neuritis:** Unlikely given the absence of pain with eye movement but should be ruled out with further imaging and assessment. Optic neuritis often

presents with painful vision loss and the individual may also have generalized demyelinating symptoms.

- **Central Retinal Artery Occlusion (CRAO):** Considered due to sudden vision loss but less likely given the absence retinal pallor and the pathognomonic cherry-red spot on macular examination. CRAO typically presents with acute, painless vision loss and these characteristic retinal findings.

Learning Points

- Identify hallmark clinical features of non-arteritic anterior ischemic optic neuropathy (NAION), including sudden painless vision loss, optic disc edema, relative afferent pupillary defect (RAPD), usually with an inferior altitudinal visual field defect. This is critical for prompt diagnosis and management.
- Understand the potential for perioperative hypotension and blood loss during surgeries such as lumbar laminectomy to precipitate NAION, or PION by compromising retrobulbar perfusion, emphasizing the importance of careful perioperative management in at-risk individuals.
- Develop a comprehensive differential diagnosis for sudden vision loss post-surgery, distinguishing between NAION and PION by recognizing the clinical features that differentiate them.
- Appreciate the importance of neuroimaging, such as MRI and MRV, in ruling out other potential etiologies of optic neuropathy such as compressive lesions or

central nervous system pathology like demyelinating disease.

Questions

What are the primary risk factors for non-arteritic anterior ischemic optic neuropathy (NAION)?

Primary risk factors for NAION in her case include hypertension, diabetes, hyperlipidemia, and perioperative hypotension. An anatomic hypoplastic optic nerve ("disc-at-risk") further increases risk.

How can NAION be differentiated from posterior ischemic optic neuropathy (PION)?

NAION typically presents with visible optic disc edema initially, whereas PION does not have visible optic neuropathy initially and requires imaging studies like MRI and MRV for diagnosis. PION is also more commonly associated with hypotension from significant blood loss during surgery.

What imaging studies are crucial for diagnosing NAION and PION?

MRI and MRV of the brain and orbits are crucial for diagnosing PION and ruling out other causes of optic neuropathy. For NAION, retinal examination and OCT are essential to assess optic nerve head changes.

Shocking

History of Present Illness (HPI)

A 39-year-old lady is in your chair after experiencing recurrent and intense shooting pain on the left side of her scalp, primarily radiating from around her eye. These episodes have increased in frequency over the past six months significantly impacting things she likes to do. Each episode is characterized by a sharp electric shock-like pain which lasts from a few seconds to several minutes. She was seen by ENT who found no abnormalities, and then referred her on to see you.

Review of Systems (ROS)

She experiences sharp shooting facial pain and occasional tingling sensations, localized mainly around her left eye and temple. She also occasionally notices some blurred vision coinciding with the pain episodes, but with no loss of vision or diplopia. She has no rashes or notable dermatologic clues in this area. She has always had a normal appetite and digestion. Most recently, she has had some difficulty sleeping.

Past Medical History (PMH)

She has generally maintained good health with no significant illnesses, surgeries, or hospitalizations. Some dental issues, including a couple root canals on her left side over the years.

Family History (FH)

Her family history is largely unremarkable. Several family members are prone to migraines.

Medications and Allergies

No prescription medication. She occasionally uses over-the-counter pain relievers but they provide minimal relief. She has no known allergies to medications, foods, or environmental factors.

Ophthalmic Examination

- **Best Corrected Visual Acuity (BCVA) :** OD 20/20, OS 20/20.
- **Pupils:** Pupils equal, round, responsive to light and accommodation. No afferent pupillary defect. PERRLA, (-)APD.
- **Extraocular Muscles (EOMs):** Full, without diplopia
- **Visual Field (VF):** Full OU.
- **Intraocular Pressure (IOP):** 18 OD, 16 OS
- **Anterior Segment:** Clear cornea, deep and quiet anterior chamber, clear lens OU.
- **Posterior Segment:** Optic nerve, macula, vessels, vitreous, retina unremarkable.
- **Optical Coherence Tomography (OCT):** Normal optic nerve and retinal nerve fiber layer (rNFL) OU, macula clear with good foveal contour OU.

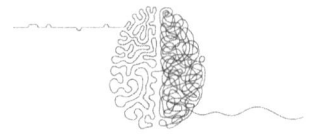

Think Deeper!

Discussion and Management

Given the severity and location of her symptoms, trigeminal neuralgia (TN), also known as "tic douloureux" is your first thought. This neuropathic disorder characterized by intense episodic facial pain aligns with her description of electric shock-like pain. It occurs along the trigeminal pathway, in her case likely the V1 distribution. You order an MRI Brain with and without contrast emphasizing the course of the trigeminal nerve, ruling-out a potential compressive source or structural abnormality which could precipitate her symptoms.

Trigeminal neuralgia is known for its sudden, severe, and debilitating facial pain. The pain typically affects one side of the face, following one of three branches of the trigeminal nerve (Vn) responsible for facial sensation. It's often described as an electric shock that can be simply triggered by things like chewing, talking, or even touching the face.

Given her intense and specific nature of the pain, you must differentiate TN from other conditions which might present with similar symptoms. These include cluster headaches, which cause severe pain around one eye and are often accompanied by tearing and nasal congestion; migraines, which can also cause severe unilateral pain but are typically accompanied by nausea, light sensitivity, and sometimes an aura; and temporomandibular joint disorders (TMJ), where problems with the jaw joint can cause pain radiating to the face.

You also consider other potential differential diagnoses include post-herpetic neuralgia, which is pain that persists after active zoster and follows a nerve distribution; multiple sclerosis, if it affects the trigeminal nerve; dental issues such as abscesses or severe tooth decay which can cause referred pain in the face; sinusitis, where inflammation of the sinuses can cause facial pain and typically accompanied by nasal symptoms; idiopathic facial pain, which is persistent facial pain without a clear underlying cause; giant cell arteritis, involving inflammation of the temporal artery typically affecting older adults causing headache and sometimes facial pain; and ear disorders such as otitis media which can also present with referred facial pain.

A thorough and systematic approach is essential to diagnose TN accurately and rule-out other potential causes. A detailed medical history, including questions regarding the nature, location, and duration of the pain; identifying trigger factors such as eating, talking, or touching the face; and reviewing any previous management is important.

Imaging studies play a key role, particularly MRI to detect structural abnormalities such as masses, vascular compression, or plaques associated with multiple sclerosis, and MRA to assess vascular integrity and identify potential vascular compression.

Regarding laboratory investigations, they are generally not specific to TN, however they will help rule out other conditions.

If you confirm trigeminal neuralgia, there are several treatment options to consider. Medications are often the first line of treatment, with anticonvulsants like carbamazepine being very effective. Other options include oxcarbazepine, gabapentin, and pregabalin. Muscle relaxants such as baclofen can also be used in conjunction with anticonvulsants, and pain management strategies might involve tricyclic antidepressants or opioids, particularly if refractory.

If she does not respond to medication, surgical approaches can be explored. Microvascular decompression (MVD) is a procedure that relieves pressure on the trigeminal nerve by moving or removing the blood vessels compressing it. This is often combined with utilizing a teflon pad to help separate and isolate the Vn. Other surgical options include radiofrequency rhizotomy which destroys some Vn fibers, and gamma knife radiosurgery which uses focused radiation to disrupt the trigeminal nerve providing pain relief.

Adjunct therapies can also play a role in managing TN, such as physical therapy to address associated muscle tension and improve overall function, and psychological support to help individuals cope with the chronic pain and its impact on what they do.

Finally, you consider vitamin B12 deficiency which can contribute to neuropathic symptoms. Checking serum B12 and folate levels is always important. A deficiency if confirmed can be managed with B12 supplementation, via oral, sublingual, or intra-muscular injections.

Differential Diagnoses and Rationale

- **Trigeminal Neuralgia:** Primary diagnosis based on the characteristic nature of her facial pain and its distribution.
- **Temporal Arteritis:** Although less common in her age group, her symptom location and severity needs to be considered. Immediate labs including ESR and CRP

are necessary, and if elevated consistent with arteritis, this is followed by a temporal artery biopsy.

- **Cluster Headaches:** Considered due to the episodic nature and severe pain localized around her eye, but the lack of autonomic symptoms such as lacrimation and conjunctival injection typically associated with cluster headaches makes this less likely.
- **Secondary Pain from Dental Origin:** Post-dental procedures, however, her ongoing symptoms supports a neuralgia diagnosis rather than dental issues.
- **Optic Neuritis:** While optic neuritis could produce similar symptoms, normal findings on OCT and lack of acute visual symptoms reduce this likelihood.
- **Herpes Zoster (Shingles):** A possibility given her age and the characteristic sharp shooting pain. Early symptoms can occur without dermatologic signs and could explain the localized neuralgic pain. Asking her to be aware of possible characteristic lesions is important.

Learning Points

- Recognize the characteristic presentation of trigeminal neuralgia, including sharp electric shock-like pain along the trigeminal nerve distribution.
- Understand the importance of MRI in ruling out compressive lesions or structural abnormalities in individuals with suspected trigeminal neuralgia.
- Emphasize the role of anticonvulsants like carbamazepine or gabapentin in managing trigeminal neuralgia and the importance of a multidisciplinary approach to care.

- Highlight the need to consider temporal arteritis in individuals with localized scalp and facial pain, especially with associated symptoms like jaw claudication and visual disturbances, and the importance of prompt evaluation and treatment.
- Appreciate the potential contribution of vitamin B12 deficiency to neurologic symptoms and the importance of checking serum B12 and folate levels in the diagnostic workup.

Questions

What imaging modality is essential for ruling out compressive lesions in individuals with trigeminal neuralgia symptoms?

MRI of the brain focusing on the trigeminal nerve distribution is essential for ruling out compressive lesions or structural abnormalities that could be precipitating trigeminal neuralgia symptoms.

What is the primary pharmacological treatment for trigeminal neuralgia and its mechanism of action?

The primary pharmacological treatment for trigeminal neuralgia is anticonvulsants such as carbamazepine or gabapentin. These medications stabilize nerve activity and reduce pain by inhibiting voltage-gated sodium channels and modulating the release of excitatory neurotransmitters.

Why should temporal arteritis be considered in patients with localized scalp and facial pain, and what are key diagnostic investigations?

Temporal arteritis should be considered due to the risk of vision loss and other serious complications if left untreated.

Key diagnostics include measuring inflammatory markers such as ESR and CRP, and if elevated obtaining a temporal artery biopsy to confirm the diagnosis.

How can vitamin B12 deficiency contribute to neurologic symptoms, and what is the preferred method of supplementation if deficiency is confirmed?

Vitamin B12 deficiency can cause neurologic symptoms such as tingling, numbness, and neuropathic pain. The preferred method of supplementation if a deficiency is confirmed includes sublingual routes or injections to ensure adequate absorption, especially if gastrointestinal absorption is compromised as in pernicious anemia or previous RnY gastric bypass. Oral B12 supplements, such as 1000mcg, can be safe and effective provided there is not a contraindication in terms of absorption ability.

What are the differential diagnoses for sharp shooting facial pain and how are they distinguished?

Differential diagnoses include trigeminal neuralgia, temporal arteritis, cluster headaches, secondary pain from dental origin, optic neuritis, and herpes zoster. They are distinguished by the clinical presentation, associated symptoms, imaging findings, and diagnostic labs such as ESR, CRP, and temporal artery biopsy.

Weigh-In

History of Present Illness (HPI)

A 49-year-old lady is in your chair for a second opinion while considering bariatric surgery, and she is very apprehensive about such a big decision. She has a strong family history of glaucoma and was told by another doctor she is "borderline". She asks you if having surgery will "help or hurt" her eyes.

Review of Systems (ROS)

Longstanding obesity. Most recently she has been having more frequent headaches, trouble breathing, difficulty sleeping, and generally fatigued during the day.

Past Medical History (PMH)

She has lifetime history of obesity with much difficulty losing weight. Hypertension and type-2 diabetes, which have also been managed poorly for many years. Recently she has been having even more difficulty keeping her blood pressure and blood glucose levels under control. Her most recent A1C was 7.9.

Family History (FH)

Type-2 diabetes, hypertension, and glaucoma in both her mother and father. Migraines are common among her relatives.

Medications and Allergies

Metformin 500mg and Lisinopril 10mg daily. She has no known allergies to medication, food, or environmental factors.

Ophthalmic Examination

- **Best Corrected Visual Acuity (BCVA):** OD 20/20, OS 20/20.

- **Pupils:** Pupils are equal, round, responsive to light and accommodation, no afferent pupillary defect. PERRLA, (-)APD.
- **Extraocular Muscles (EOMs):** Full, no diplopia
- **Visual Field (VF):** Full OU
- **Intraocular Pressure (IOP):** 14 OD, 12 OS.
- **Anterior Segment:** Clear cornea, deep and quiet anterior chamber, clear lens OU.
- **Posterior Segment:** Optic disc hypoplastic, aka "disc-at-risk" OU. Macula, vessels, vitreous, retina unremarkable OU. No evidence of diabetic or hypertensive retinopathy OU.
- **Optical Coherence Tomography (OCT):** Hypoplastic disc, borderline retinal nerve fiber layer (rNFL) thinning OU. Macula clear with good foveal contour OU.

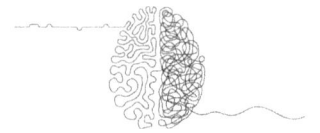

Think Deeper!

Discussion and Management

You are familiar with the various bariatric surgeries available to help individuals with obesity achieve significant weight loss, with one of the most common procedures being roux-en-y gastric bypass (RYGB). This surgery involves creating a small pouch from the stomach and connecting it directly to the small intestine, effectively bypassing a large part of the stomach and most of the small intestine. This modification reduces the amount of food that can be eaten and the absorption of nutrients.

Another popular option is the sleeve gastrectomy, where a substantial portion of the stomach is removed leaving a tube-shaped stomach about the size of a banana. This drastically limits the stomach's capacity and the physical amount of food one can consume.

Adjustable gastric banding (AGB) is also widely performed, involving the placement of a band around the upper part of the stomach to create a small pouch. The band can be adjusted by adding or removing saline through a port placed under the skin, allowing control over the size of the stomach opening.

A more complex intervention, is the biliopancreatic diversion with duodenal switch (BPD/DS). This surgery involves two steps, first a portion of the stomach is removed similar to a sleeve gastrectomy, and second the small intestine is re-routed. However, this will also separate the flow of food from bile and pancreatic enzymes thereby reducing nutrient absorption which will need compensated for.

Intragastric balloon procedures are less invasive and involve placing a deflated balloon into the stomach, which is then filled with saline. This balloon occupies space in the stomach, leading to less appetite by increasing the feeling of fullness.

Another option is the endoscopic sleeve gastroplasty (ESG), where sutures are placed in the stomach utilizing an endoscope to reduce its size and also diminishing appetite.

For your patient considering bariatric surgery, you first need to know and understand what type. You learn she is considering roux-en-y gastric bypass and fully understanding potential overall as well as ophthalmic implications is of course important.

Unlike procedures such as sleeve gastrectomy which primarily reduce stomach size, roux-en-y bypasses the stomach and small intestine which includes the duodenum, jejunum, and ileum. Intrinsic factor via gastric parietal cells which is required to bind B12 and prepare it for absorption, will essentially be non-existent. This is combined with a drastic reduction of B12 absorption capacity being it is primarily absorbed via the ileum, which will also be nearly non-existent. Additionally, it is important to note iron absorption via the duodenum will not be possible. Therefore, a combination of both iron and B12 deficiency can ensue possibly complicating her clinical course.

B12 is essential for the maintenance of myelin, our protective sheath insulating neuronal fibers which is required for proper nerve conduction. Therefore, B12 deficiency can lead to downstream neuronal demyelination and conduction deficits inducing generalized neuropathy, including optic neuropathy. Given glaucoma is fundamentally a form of optic neuropathy characterized by progressive damage, maintaining adequate levels of B12 is particularly important in prevention and management. B12 deficiency exacerbates the risk of glaucomatous optic neuropathy because it can directly impact optic nerve integrity and function, making it more susceptible to insult from other factors like intraocular pressure variations or vascular compromise and insufficiency.

Understanding her particular upcoming surgery, you know the importance of managing this risk by ensuring her post-surgical diet and supplementation is in line with the implications of roux-en-y. This usually includes lifetime regular intramuscular (IM) B12 injections. Managing her serum B12 levels regularly will be an essential part of her postoperative care to prevent deficiency and potential system wide complications, including glaucomatous optic neuropathy.

Your approach managing her concerns about glaucoma, specifically normal-tension glaucoma, should therefore prioritize neuroprotection over simple intraocular pressure reduction. This involves communicating with her family physician, and additional specialties will likely need to be on board depending on her cardiovascular status and glucose control. This is very important for maintaining optimal ocular perfusion and required nutrition so to reduce risk of progressive optic neuropathy. Thankfully, control of her hypertension and diabetes is much more likely to improve post-surgery with weight loss, diet, and exercise as recommended.

A nutritionist specializing in post-bariatric surgery should automatically be on board to develop a plan ensuring adequate nutrient and supplement intake, particularly focusing on B12, iron, calcium, and vitamin D, all of which are commonly deficient post-surgery. You also realize poor oxygen saturation, anemia, due to lack of both iron (duodenal absorption) and B12 (ileum absorption) can only further contribute to progressive glaucomatous optic neuropathy, as it may create a persistent hypoxic state.

Finally, engaging her in support groups or counseling services can help manage her stress and anxiety related to upcoming surgery and onward.

Differential Diagnoses and Rationale

- **Normal-Tension Glaucoma:** High risk given her optic disc morphology ("disc-at-risk") and medical issues related to obesity, including type-2 diabetes and hypertension. Intraocular pressure reduction is of course necessary, however, your focus is on perfusion, nutrition, and neuroprotection by managing her medical issues.
- **Nutritional Optic Neuropathy:** Ongoing management, particularly considering future nutritional deficiencies post roux-en-y surgery combined with diabetes and hypertension, will potentially compromise optic nerve integrity and function. Personalized dietary needs and intramuscular (IM) B12 supplementation is standard protocol. Oral B12 will not be effective because she will no longer have the ability for GI absorption and "first-pass" metabolism.

Learning Points

- Understand the implications of roux-en-y gastric bypass surgery on nutrient absorption and its impact on overall ocular health.
- Recognize the importance of maintaining adequate B12 levels to prevent progressive optic neuropathy,

especially in patients with a predisposition or existing glaucoma.

- Highlight the importance of regular monitoring of serum B12 levels, iron, and other nutrients post-surgery to prevent deficiencies and associated complications.
- Address the importance of stress management and psychological support in individuals preparing for major surgery to improve overall outcomes and quality of life.

Questions

How does roux-en-y gastric bypass surgery impact vitamin B12 absorption?

Roux-en-y gastric bypass surgery alters normal gastrointestinal anatomy, significantly reducing the ability to bind B12 as well as reducing the surface area for nutrient and B12 absorption in the small intestine.

Why is maintaining adequate vitamin B12 levels crucial for her?

Vitamin B12 is essential for the maintenance of myelin, the protective sheath around many nerve fibers including the optic nerve. Deficiency in B12 can lead to demyelination of the optic nerve exacerbating the risk of progressive optic neuropathy, particularly in glaucoma suspects or existing glaucoma.

What are the recommended methods for ensuring adequate vitamin B12 levels post-bariatric surgery?

Recommended methods include regular intramuscular injections depending on the severity of malabsorption. Sublingual can be considered as the next best route. Monitoring serum B12 levels over time is essential.

Quad Double Trouble

History of Present Illness (HPI)

A 25-year-old young man comes to see you after a recent accident riding his quad. He describes losing control in a deep mud-filled area, causing it to flip and trap him underneath. Incredibly, the arriving EMS vehicle also lost control and collided into the quad and him while he remained underneath. Despite his unfortunate chain of events, he remained conscious throughout the ordeal and declined immediate medical attention, after only having "some double vision". He believes his double vision has partially improved, however, as he's telling his story you notice he has a slight head tilt.

Review of Systems (ROS)

No additional signs or symptoms apart from diplopia. He denies loss of consciousness during or after the accident, no loss of vision, floaters, flashing lights, nausea, vomiting, headaches, or additional deficits. He does mention some ongoing neck pain.

Past Medical History (PMH)

He has no significant medical history.

Family History (FH)

None that he is aware of.

Medications and Allergies

No medications. No known allergies to medications, foods, or environmental factors.

Ophthalmic Examination

- **Best Corrected Visual Acuity (BCVA):** 20/20 OU.
- **Pupils:** Pupils equal, round, responsive to light and accommodation, no afferent pupillary defect. PERRLA, (-)APD.
- **Extraocular Muscles (EOMs):** Restricted depression in adduction OD.
- **Visual Field (VF):** Full OU.
- **Intraocular Pressure (IOP):** 15 mmHg OU.
- **Anterior Segment:** Clear cornea, deep and quiet anterior chamber, clear lens, no evidence of trauma OU.
- **Posterior Segment:** Optic disc, macula, vessels, vitreous, retina unremarkable OU. There is no evidence of retinal trauma, particularly berlins edema, macular edema, peripheral holes, tears, hemorrhages, or detachment OU.
- **Optical Coherence Tomography (OCT):** Normal optic nerve and retinal nerve fiber layer (rNFL) OU, macula clear with good foveal contour OU. There is no indication of disc edema OU.

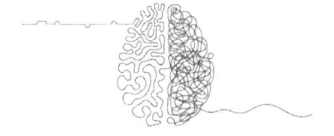

Think Deeper!

Discussion and Management

His quite unlucky traumatic chain of events necessitates your thorough and immediate work-up, and urgently with evidence of cranial nerve involvement. This is especially important considering he refused initial medical care or transportation to the ER.

You know the IV cranial nerve (trochlear) innervating the superior oblique muscle is particularly vulnerable to trauma, due to its long thin structure and unique path around the brainstem, making it susceptible to shearing forces during head trauma. Its path through the trochlear notch and posteriorly around the midbrain exposes it to potential injury from even mild to moderate head trauma. In his case, the force involved in the accident followed by secondary trauma from the EMS vehicle, likely resulted in a traction injury to the IV nerve. This will manifest as vertical and oblique diplopia, evidenced by his EOM findings, and often with a compensatory head tilt.

His classic clinical presentation of a IVn palsy includes vertical diplopia that worsens with downgaze and/or adduction. Often you will find an ipsilateral head tilt, an unconscious mechanism to compensate for ocular misalignment which will reduce diplopia. This persistent head tilt can also lead to secondary issues such as neck pain and muscle strain.

You remember the Parks-Bielschowsky three-step method, as it is a textbook diagnostic method utilized in isolating extraocular muscle palsies. However, in many cases, the nerve or muscle is obvious when truly understanding EOM anatomy and function. Just like his traumatic IVn palsy, a classic VIn palsy is also a good example of not needing to take time with the Parks method.

Of course, you cannot assume his presentation is purely an isolated traumatic IVn. Therefore, MRI with and without contrast is critical to rule-out more urgent consequences such as a traumatic epidural hematoma, subdural hematoma, brain contusion, or brainstem compression. These could not only be contributing to his IVn compromise, but instead be the primary source, potentially going on to create progressive and more severe neurologic deficits. MRI is particularly useful for evaluating soft tissue and neurologic sequela, with the "FIESTA" protocol ideal when targeting cranial nerve pathology. CT imaging is most effective for identifying hemorrhage or fractures, including an orbital "blow-out" fracture possibly restricting the superior oblique muscle.

Understanding the basis of the FIESTA protocol is important in neuro-ophthalmic diagnostics. Fast imaging employing steady-state acquisition (FIESTA) protocol is a sophisticated MRI technique which is especially effective for imaging cranial nerves. This protocol is the go-to for high resolution imaging capabilities, which are essential for visualizing the intricate details of small structures such as the cranial nerves.

FIESTA employs a balanced steady-state free precession (bSSFP) sequence, which significantly enhances the contrast between cerebrospinal fluid (CSF) and neural structures. This contrast improvement is key for clearly differentiating the cranial nerves from surrounding tissues. The technique is further distinguished by its use of three-dimensional imaging, allowing for multiplanar reconstructions and superior spatial resolution.

One of the major advantages of the FIESTA protocol is its rapid acquisition time. This speed not only improves an individual's comfort by reducing the time required to remain still during the scan, but also minimizes motion artifacts that could compromise image quality. The FIESTA protocol is invaluable for diagnosing various conditions involving any of the cranial nerves, such as trigeminal neuralgia and vestibular schwannomas.

If his diplopia becomes stable and unchanging, symptomatic management involves adding prism correction in his glasses. Prism will optically compensate for the ocular misalignment providing symptomatic relief. However, occluding or patching the affected eye is usually done first for at least one month, waiting for stability or resolution before prescribing prism.

The outcome for a traumatic IVn palsy generally depends on the severity of the injury. Some individuals experience spontaneous recovery even up to a year. If purely an isolated traumatic insult, a minimum 90-day waiting period is widely accepted for which if the diplopia continues, permanent prism or surgical correction is possible. Surgical options include recession or resection of the superior oblique tendon or weakening procedures on the antagonist muscles.

Differential Diagnoses and Rationale

- **Traumatic IV Nerve Palsy:** Primary consideration given his mechanism of injury, EOM findings, and diplopic symptoms.
- **Concussion:** Likely, considering the nature of the accident and his initial presentation with diplopia and visual disturbances.
- **Cervical Spine Injury:** Possible due to the dynamics of the accident and neck pain, requiring assessment for any potential spinal involvement.

Learning Points

- Recognize the characteristic signs and symptoms of a IVn palsy, including restricted depression in the adducted position and an ipsilateral compensatory head tilt.
- Understand the importance of a comprehensive diagnostic workup in trauma presenting with neurologic symptoms, including imaging studies and detailed neuro-ophthalmic evaluation.
- Emphasize the role of prism in managing diplopia while awaiting further diagnostic results and/or potential recovery.

Questions

What are key diagnostic investigations for identifying a IVn palsy and its underlying cause in trauma?

Diagnostics include MRI and CT neuroimaging to looking for associated traumatic brain injury (TBI), detailed neuro-ophthalmic evaluation, and comprehensive examination of all cranial nerve function.

Why is early intervention important in managing a traumatic IVn palsy?

Answer: Early intervention is critical to identify and address the underlying etiology, possibly preventing additional or future neurologic complications. Also, improving day-to-day activities via patching or prism can be extremely helpful.

How does prism help manage diplopia in a IVn palsy?

Answer: Prism can help by optically compensating for ocular misalignment eliminating diplopia, so to more easily function day to day. This correction may be permanent, or temporary while further diagnostic evaluations and/or treatment are completed to manage the underlying etiology.

What are differential diagnoses for acute diplopia following trauma, and how are they distinguished?

Answer: Differential diagnoses include a traumatic cranial nerve palsy, concussion, and/or cervical spine injury. They are distinguished by clinical presentation, associated symptoms, and diagnostic imaging investigations such as MRI and CT.

Section 3
Brain

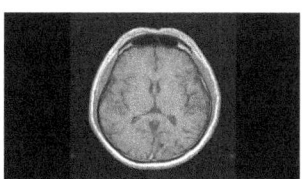

"The human brain has 100 billion neurons, each neuron connected to 10 thousand other neurons. Sitting on your shoulders is the most complicated object in the known universe."

– Dr. Michio Kaku

She Loves You

History of Present Illness (HPI)

A 25-year-old young lady is in your chair with a long history of ocular migraines, characterized by scintillating scotomas and nausea followed by intense pain. She previously came to see you as a last resort thinking perhaps her eyes or vision may be the problem. You simply suggested she begin taking magnesium supplements, and to her surprise she is feeling better than ever! Her headaches are now infrequent, the visual auras have disappeared, and no more upset stomach. She credits you and is absolutely overjoyed with gratitude for resolving her years of migraine problems, so she wonders why other doctors never mentioned a seemingly simple fix.

Review of Systems (ROS)

Only occasional nausea associated with her now less frequent headaches.

Past Medical History (PMH)

Known history of migraine headache with aura including gastrointestinal and visual symptoms.

Family History (FH)

Mother also with migraines.

Medications and Allergies

Occasional acetaminophen or ibuprofen as needed. No known allergies to medications, foods, or environmental factors.

Ophthalmic Examination

- **Best Corrected Visual Acuity (BCVA):** 20/20 OU.
- **Pupils:** Pupils equal, round, reactive to light and accommodation, no afferent pupillary defect. PERRLA, (-)APD.
- **Extraocular Muscles (EOMs):** Full, without diplopia.
- **Visual Field (VF):** Full OU.
- **Intraocular Pressure (IOP):** 21mmHg OU.
- **Anterior Segment:** Clear cornea, deep and quiet anterior chamber, clear lens OU.
- **Posterior Segment:** Optic nerve, macula, vessels, vitreous, retina unremarkable OU.

- **Optical Coherence Tomography (OCT):** Normal optic nerve and retinal nerve fiber layer (rNFL) OU, macula clear with good foveal contour OU.

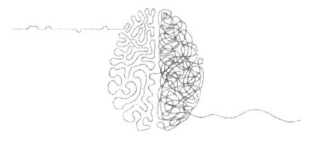

Think Deeper!

Discussion and Management

You're also amazed apparently no-one ever addressed magnesium or suggested giving it a try!

Ocular migraines involve two primary phases, the aura phase and then the pain phase, though the pain phase does not always occur. The aura phase is induced by vasospasm and/or vasoconstriction of intracranial arteries, leading to reduced cerebral blood flow and initiating what is known as cortical spreading depression (CSD). This phenomenon triggers a wave of neuronal and glial depolarization across the cortex creating the potential for a wide array of neurologic effects. Therefore, auras are not purely an ocular phenomenon, and the exact form of aura is dependent on the area of the cortex affected.

Visual auras are the most common type, often manifesting as scintillating scotomas which are flashes or flickering lights that appear in a zigzag pattern, sometimes resembling fortifications or castles. People might also experience photopsia, seeing bright spots or flashes of light, or visual field and scotoma type defects, which involve temporary loss of vision in one or both eyes that often start as a small area and expand. Also, metamorphopsia may occur causing objects to appear distorted in shape and size.

Sensory auras involve changes in sensation, such as paresthesia, which is tingling or numbness that typically begins in the fingers or hands and spreads up the arm to the face. This may also occur with a prickling sensation, often described as pins and needles and is usually unilateral.

Speech and language auras affect communication abilities, presenting as aphasia, which is difficulty in speaking or finding words, or dysphasia, an impaired ability to produce or understand speech. Motor auras, although less common, can produce hemiplegia which is temporary weakness or total paralysis on one side of the body, or ataxia which involves a lack of muscle coordination affecting movement and balance.

Brainstem auras, a rare type, involve symptoms originating from the brainstem such as vertiginous sensations, tinnitus, dysarthria which is difficulty speaking due to muscle weakness, and of course diplopia.

Olfactory and gustatory auras, also rare, include olfactory hallucinations where individuals smell odors that are not present, and gustatory hallucinations where they taste something that isn't there. These types of auras typically develop gradually over several minutes and last for about 20 to 60 minutes.

Auras are often followed by the headache pain phase, although some people may experience an aura without a subsequent headache. Understanding and recognizing these auras can help individuals manage and prepare for the onset of pain more effectively.

The pain phase, when it does occur, is generally caused by excessive rebound vasodilation. This dilatory phase increases intracranial blood flow activating trigeminal nerve pathways, leading to the release of inflammatory mediators like calcitonin gene-related peptide (CGRP), substance P, and neurokinin A, which contribute to migraine pain.

For her, magnesium played a highly therapeutic role in both preventing the initial vasoconstriction and mitigating the effects of vasodilation. By stabilizing neuronal membranes and blocking calcium influx into vascular smooth muscle, magnesium helps counteract neuronal firing and vasospasm or vasoconstriction. Understanding magnesium (Mg++) is positively charged just the same as calcium (Ca++), it will therefore "naturally" repel the unwanted calcium. Magnesium also increases nitric oxide (NO2) production present in vascular smooth muscle, creating a therapeutic dilatory effect. Additionally, this effect helps counteract the pathologic rapid rebound vascular tone which triggers migraine pain. This is why magnesium deficiency has been linked to increased neuronal excitability and vascular dysregulation, both of which are implicated in migraine pathophysiology.

Your recommended dose of 300 mg of magnesium glycinate twice daily was obviously effective and should be maintained, with adjustments as necessary based on her ongoing response and symptoms. The magnesium glycinate form is preferred due to its high bioavailability and minimal gastrointestinal side effects compared to other magnesium salts.

Finally, lifestyle changes such as maintaining a regular sleep schedule, staying hydrated, managing stress, and avoiding known migraine triggers (e.g., certain foods, caffeine, alcohol) can further reduce her frequency and severity of episodes. Other potential contributing factors such as hormonal fluctuations, dietary habits, and environmental influences are also important. Hormonal factors are particularly relevant in women of reproductive age, as fluctuations in estrogen levels during the menstrual cycle can exacerbate migraines. If you suspect a hormonal trigger, collaboration with her gynecologist may be helpful. Although her migraines are less frequent, encouraging her to keep a detailed migraine diary will aid in tracking the time, duration, and characteristics providing valuable information going forward.

In terms of pharmacological management, preventative treatments such as beta-blockers (e.g., propranolol), antiepileptic drugs (e.g., topiramate), and tricyclic antidepressants (e.g., amitriptyline) are common therapies. For acute migraine attacks, triptans (e.g., sumatriptan) or non-steroidal anti-inflammatory drugs (NSAIDs) can be effective in providing relief.

Differential Diagnoses and Rationale

- **Ocular Migraines:** Primary diagnosis supported by her symptoms and response to magnesium. Ocular migraines typically present with visual auras and are often followed by headache, although the pain phase does not always occur.

- **Cluster Headaches:** Considered but less likely due to the presence of visual aura. Cluster headaches typically do not induce a visual aura and are characterized by severe, unilateral pain around the eye, accompanied by autonomic symptoms such as tearing, nasal congestion, and/or ptosis.
- **Temporal Arteritis:** Unlikely given her age and symptoms. Temporal arteritis is more common in individuals over the age of 50 and present with symptoms such as jaw claudication, scalp tenderness, and elevated inflammatory markers such as ESR and CRP.

Learning Points

- Understand the pathophysiology of ocular migraines, including the role of cortical spreading depression and the neurovascular mechanisms involved in the aura and pain phases.
- Recognize the importance of magnesium in stabilizing neuronal membranes and displacing calcium to prevent vasospasm, as well as reducing the painful rebound dilatory phase. Know its role in migraine prophylaxis.
- Emphasize the need for a comprehensive approach to migraine management, including lifestyle changes, pharmacologic treatments, and regular follow-ups.
- Consider the impact of hormonal fluctuations and other potential triggers in women of reproductive age with migraines.
- Highlight the value of a detailed migraine diary in

tracking symptom patterns to help future treatment decisions.

Questions

What are key mechanisms involved in the pathophysiology of ocular migraines?

Mechanisms include cortical spreading depression (CSD), which triggers a wave of neuronal and glial depolarization across the cortex leading to visual auras. The pain phase when it occurs, is caused by excessive rebound vasodilation and activation of trigeminal nerve sensory pathways, resulting in the release of inflammatory cytokines and pain.

How does magnesium supplementation help in the management of migraines?

Magnesium helps stabilize neuronal membranes and block calcium influx, preventing neuronal firing and vasospasm. Its effect also lessons rapid dilatory changes in vascular tone, therefore reducing the frequency and severity of both the aura and pain phase in migraine.

What are the differential diagnoses for ocular migraines and how are they distinguished?

Differential diagnoses include cluster headaches, which typically do not involve visual auras but present with severe unilateral pain around the eye and autonomic symptoms. Also temporal arteritis, which is more common in individuals over 50 and can present with jaw claudication, temple and scalp tenderness, with elevated inflammatory markers, specifically ESR.

What role does a migraine diary play in managing migraines?

A migraine diary helps track the frequency, duration, and characteristics of migraines, providing valuable information for identifying triggers, assessing treatment effectiveness, and making informed decisions about ongoing management.

Moldy Weed

History of Present Illness (HPI)

A 29-year-old young man comes to see you because he has been having intermittent episodes of feeling dizzy and his vision "going black" while working out at his local gym. The episodes are brief and usually with complete loss of vision in both eyes, anywhere from a few seconds to approximately a minute. He also tells you about coughing up a "black substance" in the mornings, which he thinks is from smoking old "moldy weed."

Review of Systems (ROS)

He has occasional chest tightness and palpitations during these transient episodes. He denies any additional signs or symptoms such as fever, weight loss, or night sweats.

Past Medical History (PMH)

Unremarkable medical history. His last physical examination was in high school.

Family History (FH)

Father with hypertension and hyperlipidemia. Mother deceased in a motor vehicle accident with no known medical history.

Medications and Allergies

No medications, however, his diet consists mainly of "protein shakes". He has no known allergies to medication, food, or environmental factors.

Ophthalmic Examination

- **Best Corrected Visual Acuity (BCVA):** 20/20 OU.
- **Pupils:** Pupils equal, round, responsive to light and accommodation, no afferent pupillary defect. PERRLA, (-)APD.
- **Extraocular Muscles (EOMs):** Full, without diplopia.
- **Visual Field (VF):** Full OU
- **Intraocular Pressure (IOP):** 21mmHg OD, 20mmHg OS.
- **Anterior Segment:** Cornea clear, anterior chamber deep and quiet, clear lens OU.
- **Posterior Segment:** Optic nerve, macula, vessels, vitreous, retina, unremarkable OU.
- **Optical Coherence Tomography (OCT):** Normal optic nerve and retinal nerve fiber layer (rNFL) OU, macula clear with good foveal contour OU.

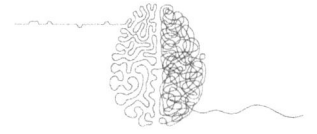

Think Deeper!

Discussion and Management

His occurrences of vertiginous symptoms with bilateral transient vision loss at the gym, which he describes as "blackouts", immediately raises your concern of the many underlying cardiovascular possibilities. However, one is at the top of your list which must be considered and ruled-out before assuming any less ominous etiologies. You therefore immediately order an ECG, Echo, carotid duplex, as well as specific labs.

Your top priority is to investigate the possibility of hypertrophic obstructive cardiomyopathy (HOCM), which is well known to create exercise-induced pre-syncope or syncope. HOCM is a genetic heart condition characterized by abnormal hypertrophy or thickening of the cardiac musculature, particularly the interventricular septum, which is the wall separating the left and right ventricles. This excessive hypertrophic state can anatomically obstruct blood flow out of the left ventricle, leading to increased cardiac workload, decreased cardiac output, with potential severe complications.

Individuals with HOCM can experience symptoms such as chest pain, dyspnea, palpitations, and syncope, especially during physical activity. It can also lead to dangerous arrhythmias, and in severe cases even sudden cardiac death, particularly in young athletes.

The diagnosis of HOCM is typically via echocardiography (Echo) which will reveal hypertrophied ventricular musculature as well as the extent of obstruction. Genetic testing is utilized to identify specific mutations associated with the disorder, as well as raising awareness for family members.

Regarding management, first line treatment involves medical therapy. Beta-blockers like propranolol and metoprolol are commonly used to reduce heart rate and myocardial contractility, which helps to decrease the obstruction and alleviate symptoms of chest pain and dyspnea. Calcium channel blockers such as verapamil and diltiazem serve a similar purpose by relaxing cardiac musculature and improving blood flow. For those experiencing arrhythmias, antiarrhythmic drugs including amiodarone or disopyramide may be used, and anticoagulants might be necessary for individuals with an increased risk of thrombus formation if atrial fibrillation.

Anyone diagnosed with HOCM is of course required to avoid strenuous physical activity, in particular competitive sports to reduce risk of cardiac events, which again includes the real possibility of sudden death. Maintaining proper hydration is also very important, as dehydration can exacerbate cardiac dysfunction.

Rarely, surgical or interventional procedures may be required. A septal myectomy involves surgically removing a portion of the hypertrophied septal wall, which can significantly improve blood flow. Alternatively, alcohol septal ablation, a less invasive procedure uses alcohol injections to shrink the thickened ventricular septum reducing obstruction.

Individuals with high risk of sudden cardiac death, an implantable cardioverter-defibrillator (ICD) may be implanted. In some cases, a dual-chamber pacemaker might be used to help coordinate the timing of contractions between the atria and ventricles, thereby reducing obstruction and improving symptoms.

His issue of coughing up a "black substance" requires you to also coordinate a proper pulmonary assessment. If truly smoking "moldy weed", it is essentially the inhalation of fungal spores and other contaminants. Serious fungal pulmonary sequela such as aspergillosis, chronic obstructive pulmonary disease (COPD), and others will only exacerbate pre-existing HOCM. Therefore, CT chest also needs to be obtained and likely a pulmonology consult.

You understand in his clinical scenario, the possibility of both hypertrophic obstructive cardiomyopathy (HOCM) and chronic obstructive pulmonary disease (COPD), an interplay of cardiovascular and respiratory dysfunction is a real possibility. This can then give rise to complex symptoms such as his bilateral vision loss and vertiginous symptoms. Bilateral temporary loss of vision can be attributed to transient ischemia/transient ischemic attacks (TIA's) resulting from decreased vertebrobasilar perfusion to the brain and occipital/visual cortex due to reduced cardiac output. COPD can also exacerbate the situation by creating hypoxemia, a state of low blood oxygen saturation which only further compromises oxygen delivery to the visual cortex. Vertiginous symptoms, or sensations of dizziness and spinning can occur for the same reasons. This affected area of the brain is the vestibular system which includes parts of the brainstem and cerebellum.

Finally, both a hypoxic and ischemic state may also impair autonomic nervous system function which regulates blood pressure and heart rate, potentially leading to further episodes of vision loss and/or vertiginous symptoms.

Differential Diagnoses and Rationale

- **Hypertrophic Obstructive Cardiomyopathy (HOCM):** Must first be investigated given the exercise-induced nature of his visual and physical symptoms. HOCM can cause transient vision loss, diplopia, pre-syncope, syncope, and even sudden cardiac death during exertion.
- **Arrhythmia:** Particularly if his vision loss is related to transient cardiac rhythm disturbances. Arrhythmias can lead to inadequate cerebral perfusion, resulting in transient vision loss or blackouts.
- **Vasovagal Syncope:** This common form of fainting can occur in response to intense emotional stress or physical triggers, such as standing for long periods or exposure to heat. It is characterized by a sudden drop in heart rate and blood pressure, leading to decreased cerebral perfusion.
- **Orthostatic Hypotension:** Some individuals may experience drops in blood pressure during exercise, leading to transient inadequate cerebral perfusion.

This condition is more common in individuals with autonomic dysfunction or volume depletion.

- **Subclavian Steal Syndrome:** This occurs when stenosis of the subclavian artery creates a reversal of blood flow in the vertebral artery during arm activity, like working out. It can lead to symptoms of dizziness, visual disturbances, and syncope during exercise.
- **Pulmonary Disease:** Likely, considering his cough and substance use history. Chronic respiratory conditions or acute infection could contribute to his symptoms.
- **Primary Pulmonary Hypertension:** Elevated pulmonary artery pressure can severely affect cardiac output during exercise, leading to pre-syncope or syncope.
- **Toxic Inhalation:** Smoking "moldy weed" could lead to inhalation of harmful substances and toxins, creating pulmonary complications and potentially affecting cardiovascular function.

Learning Points

- Understand the importance of a comprehensive cardiovascular evaluation in patients presenting with exercise induced visual disturbances, vision loss, pre-syncope or syncope.
- Recognize the potential impact of smoking and inhalation of toxic substances on pulmonary, respiratory, and cardiovascular function.
- Highlight the role of advanced imaging techniques, such as Echo and CT, in identifying underlying cardiovascular and pulmonary conditions.

- Appreciate the importance of toxicology screening in evaluating individuals with potential exposure to harmful substances.

Questions

What are key mechanisms by which hypertrophic obstructive cardiomyopathy (HOCM) can lead to vision loss, pre-syncope, or syncope during exercise?

This can occur due to the physical obstruction of blood flow from thickened septal ventricular musculature, decreased cardiac output, and possible arrhythmias triggered by physical exertion.

How can smoking "moldy weed" affect his respiratory and cardiovascular health?

Smoking "moldy weed" can lead to inhalation of fungal spores and other toxic contaminants, possibly creating pulmonary infection and pneumonia, chronic obstructive pulmonary disease (COPD), potentially impacting oxygen saturation as well as cardiovascular function.

What are some differential diagnoses for exercise induced pre-syncope or syncope, and how are they distinguished?

This can include HOCM, arrhythmia, vasovagal syncope, orthostatic hypotension, subclavian steal syndrome, pulmonary disease, primary pulmonary hypertension, and toxic inhalation. They are distinguished by clinical presentation, associated symptoms, imaging findings, and diagnostic investigations such as ECG, Echo, and toxicology screening.

Painful Blur

History of Present Illness (HPI)

A 32-year-old lady comes to see you with persistent and escalating headaches over the previous year. Her symptoms have progressively worsened to a point that she called your office to be seen as quickly as possible. She tells you around the same time as her headaches, her vision also seems to fluctuate and blur. Of course, your first question to her is if her vision (or section of vision) is "blacking out" or purely "blurred". She believes it is just blurred without any actual loss.

Review of Systems (ROS)

She has been having increasingly frequent episodes of transient visual obscurations and occasional diplopia. Her changes in vision often correlate with her headache episodes. She also tells you about a pulsatile type tinnitus with vertiginous symptoms that come and go, which seem to only exacerbate her vision issues.

Past Medical History (PMH)

She has a history of chronic headaches, previously diagnosed as recurrent migraine headaches which have recently become more frequent and severe. She is mildly obese but has no significant past medical history including diabetes, hypertension, or autoimmune disorders.

Family History (FH)

Her mother and sister both have a long history of migraine headache and hypertension. Father with hypertension, hyperlipidemia, and glaucoma.

Medications and Allergies

No medications and she recently stopped taking oral contraceptives. She has no known allergies to medications or environmental factors.

Ophthalmic Examination

- **Best Corrected Visual Acuity (BCVA)**: 20/40 OD, 20/50 OS.
- **Pupils**: Pupils equal, round, reactive to light and accommodation, no afferent pupillary defect. PERRLA, (-)APD.
- **Extraocular Muscles (EOMs)**: Full, no diplopia.
- **Visual Field (VF)**: Enlarged blind spot OU.
- **Intraocular Pressure (IOP)**: 21 OD, 22 OS.
- **Anterior Segment**: Clear cornea, deep and quiet anterior chamber, clear lens OU.
- **Posterior Segment**: Optic nerve with significant disc edema OU. Macula, vessels, vitreous, retina unremarkable.
- **Optical Coherence Tomography (OCT)**: Shows bilateral disc edema indicative of papilledema OU. Macula clear with good foveal contour OU.

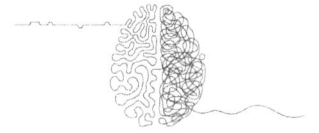

Think Deeper!

Discussion and Management

Understanding the possible differentials, some of which could be quite ominous or urgent, you immediately order an MRI/MRV Brain with and without contrast. Her imaging reveals bilateral optic nerve sheath tortuosity, a partial sella, and evidence of dural venous sinus thrombosis (DVST). You know these findings all underscore increased cerebral spinal fluid (CSF) pressure and intracranial pressure (ICP). Her optic nerve sheath tortuosity is particularly significant, as it often correlates with elevated intracranial pressure frequently found in pseudotumor cerebri or idiopathic intracranial hypertension (IIH). The imaging finding of a partial or empty sella also raises your degree of suspicion for IIH, though it does not alone confirm the diagnosis.

In IIH, increased intracranial pressure can force CSF into the suprasellar space, potentially compressing the pituitary gland and resulting in an imaging appearance and finding known as partial or empty sella. However, this radiologic sign is not exclusive to IIH and can be incidentally found in individuals undergoing MRI for unrelated reasons. Despite its ominous appearance, it is interesting to note many individuals with partial or empty sella syndrome maintain normal pituitary function and hormone balance.

Further supporting your suspicion of pseudotumor cerebri, DVST is found in a significant portion of these individuals with studies indicating its presence in over 90% of cases. Similarly to a partial or empty sella, the presence of DVST by itself also does not clinch a diagnosis of IIH as it can manifest in other conditions including coagulopathies or as an isolated idiopathic finding. The dural venous sinuses serve as major conduits for CSF outflow, interfacing with the subarachnoid space via one-way arachnoid granulations and facilitating drainage through both superficial and deep cerebral venous pathways. It is postulated that dysfunctional arachnoid granulations may impede CSF outflow, thus elevating intracranial pressure and contributing to the development of IIH. Given these dynamics, the etiology of DVST always needs to be further considered and investigated. Structural anomalies, various coagulopathic states impeding venous and CSF drainage, or from venous stasis secondary to defective granulations all are on the differential.

The gold standard for diagnosing IIH is lumbar puncture, which will demonstrate elevated CSF pressure typically greater than 15mmHg in a lateral decubitus position and with normal CSF composition. This finding coupled with the clinical and radiologic evidence, solidifies your diagnosis of IIH.

Management requires a nuanced approach, beginning with an endocrine evaluation which includes a full assessment of pituitary function, complete labs including coagulation and lipid panel, pregnancy screening and history, as well as investigations with respect to polycystic ovarian syndrome (PCOS). PCOS and increased BMI/obesity are notoriously linked to pseudotumor cerebri.

Key management involves weight reduction strategies even in mildly obese patients, as weight loss has been shown to significantly reduce intracranial pressure in IIH. Diuretic medications such as acetazolamide, a carbonic anhydrase inhibitor (CAI), are often prescribed to increase diuresis and decrease CSF production thereby lowering intracranial pressure. In cases where acetazolamide is insufficient or not tolerated, other diuretics like furosemide may be considered. For individuals with refractory symptoms or progressive visual loss, surgical interventions such as optic nerve sheath fenestration or a cerebrospinal fluid ventriculoperitoneal (VP) or lumboperitoneal (LP) shunt may be necessary.

Your vigilance is needed to be aware of the not uncommon prevalence of IIH in certain demographics, to prevent a common misdiagnosis of "migraine", and to ensure treatment is both appropriate and effective. Proper management will mitigate risks such as irreversible optic atrophy and permanent vision loss. A multidisciplinary approach involving neurology and possibly neurosurgery is essential for managing these sometimes complex scenarios.

Differential Diagnoses and Medical Rationale

- **Idiopathic Intracranial Hypertension (IIH)/Pseudotumor Cerebri**: Strongly supported by her combination of clinical signs and symptoms, imaging findings of optic nerve sheath tortuosity, partial sella, and dural venous sinus thrombosis, then corroborated by lumbar puncture results.

- **Dural Venous Sinus Thrombosis (DVST)**: Present in the imaging, it can be a primary complicating factor or a secondary effect of elevated intracranial pressure in IIH.
- **Secondary Causes of Intracranial Hypertension**: Considered given her spectrum of symptoms and findings but less likely due to the absence of structural lesions or contributing findings on imaging. She also lacks a relevant medical history which could predispose her to other etiologies inducing IIH.

Learning Points

- Recognize the characteristic symptoms and signs of idiopathic intracranial hypertension (IIH) such as headaches, transient visual obscurations, pulsatile tinnitus, and papilledema.
- Understand the importance of MRI and MRV in visualizing structural abnormalities and/or vascular pathology that support a diagnosis of IIH.
- Emphasize the role of lumbar puncture in confirming elevated CSF pressure and solidifying a diagnosis of IIH.
- Highlight the initial management strategies for IIH, including weight reduction and medical therapy with diuretics like acetazolamide, and the indications for surgical interventions in refractory cases.

Questions

What imaging findings are suggestive of idiopathic intracranial hypertension (IIH)?

Imaging findings suggestive of IIH include bilateral optic nerve sheath tortuosity, a partial or empty sella, and dural venous sinus thrombosis.

What is the gold standard for diagnosing IIH and why?

The gold standard for diagnosing IIH is lumbar puncture that demonstrates elevated CSF pressure greater than 15mmHg in a lateral decubitus position, with otherwise normal CSF composition.

How does acetazolamide help in the management of IIH?

Acetazolamide is a carbonic anhydrase inhibitor that reduces CSF production and increases diuresis, thereby lowering intracranial pressure decreasing or eliminating compressive neuropathology and symptoms of IIH.

What are potential complications of untreated IIH?

This includes irreversible compressive optic neuropathy and atrophy leading to possible permanent vision loss, as well as chronic headache and/or other neurologic complications due to sustained elevated intracranial pressure.

Mysterious Loss

History of Present Illness (HPI)

A 49-year-old lady is in your chair experiencing transient complete loss of vision, with two episodes approximately six months apart. Her first episode occurred in her left eye and the second involved both eyes, each lasting one or two minutes. She describes these events as sudden and total with no associated pain, preceding aura, or other signs or symptoms before, during, or after this happens.

Review of Systems (ROS)

During the past several months, she occasionally experiences vertiginous symptoms, particularly when changing positions. She tells you about feeling off-balance and sometimes needs to hold onto furniture to steady herself when she stands up quickly. She also mentions a general feeling of fatigue, and feels like she is not sleeping despite trying to get an adequate number of hours per night. She has no recent changes in weight, appetite, or diet.

Past Medical History (PMH)

A recent CT scan ordered by her family physician showed no abnormalities. She has no significant medical history and has not been on long-term medication. Her physical exam and labs, including a complete blood count (CBC), comprehensive metabolic panel (CMP), and thyroid function tests were also unremarkable. She has no history of cardiovascular disease, diabetes, or neurologic disorders. She was therefore given the assumed diagnosis of vertigo, and suggested she follow-up with ENT.

Family History (FH)

Both her parents had hypertension and hyperlipidemia, with her father having a stroke in his early 60s. There is no family history of migraines, seizures, or neurologic conditions.

Medications and Allergies

She is not taking any medications and has no known allergies to medications, foods, or environmental factors.

Ophthalmic Examination:

- **Best Corrected Visual Acuity (BCVA):** 20/20 OU.
- **Pupils:** Pupils equal, round, reactive to light and accommodation, no afferent pupillary defect. PERRLA, (-)APD.
- **Extraocular Muscles (EOMs):** Full, without diplopia.
- **Visual Field (VF):** Full OU.
- **Intraocular Pressure (IOP):** 12 mmHg OD, 13 mmHg OS.
- **Anterior Segment:** Clear cornea, deep and quiet anterior chamber, clear lens OU.
- **Posterior Segment:** Optic nerve, macula, vessels, vitreous, retina unremarkable OU.
- **Optical Coherence Tomography (OCT):** Normal optic nerve and retinal nerve fiber layer (rNFL) OU, macula clear with good foveal contour OU.

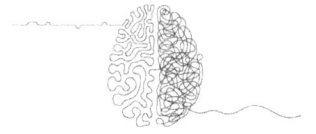

Think Deeper!

Discussion and Management

Her presentation of complete transient unilateral and bilateral vision loss, with no significant past medical history or ongoing medication, puts you in a position to coordinate an urgent cardiovascular and neurologic work-up. This is despite her being cleared by previous doctors, because you know to assume nothing. Vertigo is not a medical rationale or source of vision loss. Her symptoms, particularly given their transient nature and association with positional changes, could suggest a missed cardiovascular etiology such as carotid or vertebrobasilar insufficiency, or perhaps a primary cardiac source. You also consider a complex migraine variant.

Your understanding of the importance of not assuming "vertigo" is paramount. Therefore, additional important diagnostic investigations must be pursued. This includes carotid duplex assessing potential stenosis and associated vascular insufficiency, and/or atherosclerotic emboli risk which can present with transient unilateral or bilateral visual field defects, even possibly amaurosis fugax. An echocardiogram is imperative in terms of a potential cardiac valvular source of atherosclerotic emboli. Similarly, atrial fibrillation and other arrhythmias can lead to the formation of thrombotic emboli which of course can also travel into the cerebral circulation. Therefore an ECG is also indicated, however, if her ECG is normal then 24-hour Holter monitoring over a period of two weeks is warranted looking for intermittent cardiac arrhythmias, which may not be present at the time of an "on the fly" ECG. Standard ECG is only representative of cardiac status over a few minutes. You know these forms and sources of emboli are not uncommon, and transient ischemic attacks (TIAs) can present with purely isolated ocular symptoms.

Given her poor sleep, you also consider the possibility of an element of sleep apnea. Central or obstructive sleep apnea (OSA) can contribute to daytime somnolence from widespread hypoxia by its effect on cerebral oxygen perfusion. At the same time, reduced oxygen perfusion can potentially induce transient visual disturbances whether it be via cerebral or ocular hypoxia. Additionally, it is important to consider her symptoms in the context of migraine variants. Migrainous aura's, specifically retinal or ophthalmic migraines, can present with transient loss of vision and are often associated with other migraine symptoms including dizziness and/or sleep disturbances. A detailed headache history and assessment for migraine triggers and patterns can be helpful for her.

Management strategies involve a multidisciplinary approach, incorporating insights from cardiology, neurology, and possibly sleep medicine. Neurology consult is essential to evaluate for central causes of her visual symptoms, such as migraine variants mentioned. Carotid artery disease or other vascular pathology may require intervention, such as medical management with anticoagulation or anti-platelet therapy as well as surgical intervention if significant stenosis is discovered. Carotid endarterectomy (CEA) of course can be lifesaving. Cardiology on board to assess for various arrhythmias, cardiomyopathy, valvular disease, and other sources possibly contributing to her issues. The potential diagnosis and treatment of sleep apnea should not be overlooked. Continuous positive airway pressure (CPAP) therapy or other therapies could alleviate her symptoms and likely improve the daily fatigue she feels.

Her scenario underscores the importance of a thorough and systematic approach to transient visual disturbances. Her combination of transient loss of vision, vertiginous symptoms, and sleep disturbances, with no significant past medical history suggests an interplay of vascular, neurologic, and possibly sleep-related factors. Your multidisciplinary approach involving detailed diagnostic evaluations and targeted management strategies is key to address her symptoms effectively and solve her puzzle.

Differential Diagnoses and Medical Rationale

- **Vertebrobasilar Insufficiency:** Her simultaneous and bilateral transient visual disturbances including vertiginous symptoms could suggest reduced blood flow and perfusion within the posterior circulation, which also supplies the occipital lobe and visual cortex.
- **Carotid Artery Disease:** Internal carotid stenosis can reduce blood flow and perfusion to the brain, optic nerve via the ophthalmic artery, and retinal vasculature leading to temporary vision loss, especially with positional changes. Atherosclerotic embolic plaques (Hollenhorst plaques) can oftentimes be found lodged in retinal arteriolar bifurcations leading to permanent visual field defects as in a branch retinal artery occlusion (BRAO), or a more devastating central retinal artery occlusion (CRAO) resulting in severe vision loss. Carotid artery disease is very often found with coronary artery disease.
- **Cardiac Arrhythmias:** Various arrhythmias, such as very common atrial fibrillation, can lead to reduced

cardiac output, hemodynamic instability, blood pressure variations also affecting cerebral and/or ocular perfusion. Transient (TIAs) or permanent visual disturbances (stroke) such as hemianopic visual field defects or cranial nerve palsies with resultant diplopia are not uncommon. Thromboemboli form during arrhythmic episodes by blood "pooling" in the atria and can find their way anywhere, leading to ischemic stroke and/or brainstem infarct. Also keep in mind with coexisting valvular disease, the risk of cardiac atheroemboli being released is increased.

- **Migraine Variants:** Migrainous visual auras or disturbances, including retinal migraines or ocular migraines, can present with monocular of binocular transient loss of vision and can also be associated with vertiginous symptoms and sleep disturbances.

- **Sleep Apnea:** Obstructive sleep apnea creating pulmonary hypoxemia can contribute to widespread hypoxia and cerebral hypoperfusion, inducing transient visual symptoms and/or daytime fatigue. Transient loss of vision, monocular or binocular visual field obscurations, visual aura's, and diplopia can be more likely to occur with reduced oxygen saturation.

Learning Points

- Recognize the importance of considering cardiovascular etiologies, such as vertebrobasilar insufficiency and/or carotid artery disease in individuals with transient visual disturbances.
- Understand the role of migraine variants, including ocular and retinal migraines in causing transient

visual symptoms and associated vertiginous symptoms.

- Highlight the need for a comprehensive cardiovascular evaluation, including carotid duplex, ECG, Echo, as well as Holter monitoring to identify possible carotid stenosis, arrhythmias, and/or valvular disease contributing to visual disturbances.
- Emphasize the importance of sleep studies in evaluating individuals with sleep disturbances and transient visual symptoms, particularly for diagnosing obstructive sleep apnea.

Questions

What role does carotid duplex play in evaluating her transient visual disturbances?

Carotid duplex assesses for carotid artery disease or stenosis, which can present with permanent or transient loss of vision like monocular amaurosis fugax, as well as monocular or binocular visual field deficits due to reduced ocular and/or cerebral perfusion.

Why is an echocardiogram important in her evaluation?

An echocardiogram helps identify a potential cardiac source of valvular atherosclerotic emboli, which could result in permanent or transient visual disturbances. Conditions like atrial fibrillation found on ECG can lead to atrial thromboemboli formation or trigger the release of atheroemboli, both of which can be visualized on echo.

How might cardiac arrhythmias contribute to her symptoms?

Cardiac arrhythmias discovered via ECG can lead to hemodynamic instability which includes fluctuations in cardiac output and blood pressure, affecting cerebral perfusion and potentially leading to vertiginous episodes and/or visual disturbances. Thromboemboli may also form and be released compromising cerebral and/or ocular perfusion.

What is the significance of a sleep study in her evaluation?

A sleep study will evaluate for clinical signs of obstructive sleep apnea which can contribute to hypoxemia, widespread hypoxia, resulting in generalized cerebral oxygen hypoperfusion. Transient symptoms can include vision loss, visual field obscurations, diplopia, visual auras, as well as daytime fatigue being more likely to occur due to poor oxygen saturation.

How can migraine variants create transient loss of vision?

Migraine variants, including ocular and retinal migraines, can be a source of transient visual aura's, scintillating scotomas, visual field deficits, and on rare occasions permanent vision or visual field loss. This is directly related to cerebral vasospasm and vasoconstriction occurring during the initial phase of migraine, creating transient or sometimes permanent ischemic events.

Blotchy Vision

History of Present Illness (HPI)

A 66-year-old gentleman is referred to you by his family physician after noticing a "section of vision missing", and needs your opinion regarding a pituitary cystic lesion he was diagnosed with three months prior to seeing you. He has a neurologist on board following him as well. He describes his change in vision as a persistent "blotch" just off center to the right, in his right eye.

Review of Systems (ROS)

He has no additional signs or symptoms potentially correlating with his vision loss, which he believes was rather sudden. He has occasional unilateral headaches which are most often on his left side which he feels is "nothing new".

Past Medical History (PMH)

Apart from a recently diagnosed pituitary lesion, his medical history is relatively unremarkable. He only recently began seeing a family physician and now neurology. He believes he has been in good health over the years.

Family History (FH)

He has no significant family history that he can recall, including neurologic or ocular conditions.

Medications and Allergies

No medications and he has no known allergies to medications or environmental factors.

Ophthalmic Examination

- **Best Corrected Visual Acuity (BCVA):** 20/25 OD

with the presence of the described "blotch",
20/20 OS.

- **Pupils:** Pupils equal, round, reactive to light and accommodation, no afferent pupillary defect. PERRLA, (-)APD.
- **Extraocular Muscles (EOMs):** Full, without diplopia.
- **Visual Field (VF):** Relatively non-congruous right homonymous hemianopia.
- **Intraocular Pressure (IOP):** 14 mmHg OU.
- **Anterior Segment:** Clear cornea, deep and quiet anterior chamber, early nuclear lens changes OU.
- **Posterior Segment:** Optic nerve, macula, vessels, vitreous, retina unremarkable OU. No evidence of disc edema OU.
- **Optical Coherence Tomography (OCT):** Normal optic nerve and retinal nerve fiber layer (rNFL) OU, macula clear with good foveal contour OU.

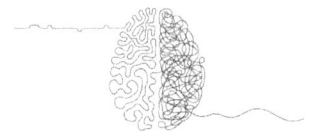

Think Deeper!

Discussion and Management

You assume nothing and know it is crucial to explore beyond his presenting diagnosis of a pituitary lesion, and not be swayed to automatically expect pituitary compression and mass effect.

Believing you will find a textbook bi-temporal hemianopic visual field defect is not your initial approach, for several reasons, and primarily because his vision loss was sudden.

His visual field defect, specifically a right homonymous hemianopia, indicates neurologic involvement beyond the anterior visual pathway and optic chiasm instead implicating the optic tract, radiations, or occipital lobe. The pattern of his visual field defect suggests a left-sided post-chiasmal lesion, and while the pituitary lesion could be implicated, other sources must be considered. His description of a "blotch" in his vision occurring rather suddenly, combined with a non-congruous right homonymous hemianopia, of course raises your suspicion of an acute vascular event. Congruity gives a clue as to the anatomic location, if very congruous and symmetric the area in question is most like farther posterior, close to or within the occipital cortex. If less congruous as in his case, it will be more anterior such as in the optic tract or radiations.

Your understanding of the dynamics of pituitary cystic lesions, reviewing or repeating neuroimaging with greater emphasis on the optic chiasm and surrounding structures is a priority. Your concern is that while the lesion is described as pituitary, its effect on the visual pathway must be delineated clearly looking for compression or secondary inflammation creating an atypical presentation. Pituitary lesions often affect the optic chiasm leading to a bitemporal hemianopia, however, atypical growth patterns or large lesions could extend to involve the optic tracts resulting in homonymous visual field deficits.

Your collaboration and communication with neurology is therefore essential to understand his complete picture and possibly switch gears in terms of etiology. Neurology can provide expertise in determining if the lesion's location correlates with the visual field defect or if an alternative cerebral pathology exists, which in his case is more characteristic of an ischemic infarct or stroke. Additional investigations, including advanced MRI techniques or CT angiography may be needed to further assess for vascular anomalies or other intracranial pathologies to better explain his sudden homonymous visual field defect. Just as you did not assume pituitary mass effect, you do not assume stroke until all possibilities are ruled-out.

Your immediate management includes neuroprotective strategies, in his case meaning medical and/or surgical indications to treat and manage an identifiable source. Medical management of suspected vascular events includes maintaining optimal blood pressure control, ensuring good glycemic control, addressing any lipid abnormalities, as well as investigating and following his cardiac status.

His occasional headaches cannot be dismissed, particularly in the context of his pituitary lesion and vision loss. Managing any change in the pattern or severity of his headaches is important, as this could indicate increasing intracranial pressure or other complications related to his pituitary lesion. It is also possible his headaches were arteritic increasing risk of stroke. His lab results including ESR and CRP need to be reviewed, and if not previously obtained, now ordered.

His visual field defect must be closely tracked over time. Some resolution is in line with stroke recovery, however, progression is more ominous pointing to a compressive or mass effect source. Repeat OCT's are also very important with respect to possible increasing intracranial pressure, with progressive papilledema, and/or long-term ischemia or ischemic events leading to related optic neuropathy.

Pituitary lesions, particularly cystic ones, can vary in their impact on the visual pathways. While they typically create a bitemporal hemianopia, unusual growth patterns can affect other parts of the visual pathway leading to atypical visual field defects and/or increasing intracranial pressure. Of course, endocrinology needs to also be on board to more closely evaluate his pituitary function. This is to specifically manage potential hormone alterations and balance from compression of tissue, and/or a hormonally active cystic adenoma. The most common active adenoma is a prolactinoma, for which multiple downstream effects are possible such as amenorrhea in women or gynecomastia in men. Medical treatment options such as bromocriptine, a dopamine agonist inhibiting prolactin production may be used to control dysregulation. Surgical intervention and resection may also be indicated.

In terms of surgical management, transsphenoidal surgery is a common approach for pituitary adenomas, especially when creating significant compression of the optic chiasm or other adjacent structures. This minimally invasive surgery involves accessing the pituitary gland through the nasal cavity, allowing for the removal of the lesion with reduced recovery time compared to traditional open surgery. Although transsphenoidal surgery has proven to be very successful, cerebrospinal fluid leaks and/or additional hormonal dysregulation is always a possibility post-operatively.

Overall, his management requires a comprehensive multidisciplinary approach involving endocrinology, cardiology, neurology, and possibly neurosurgery. Your recommendation of serial OCT's and visual fields, regular neuroimaging, and addressing vascular risk factors are part of this management.

Differential Diagnoses and Medical Rationale

- **Stroke:** Considering his sudden vision loss and the pattern of his visual field, an acute ischemic cerebral vascular event is the top differential. A stroke along the optic tract, optic radiations, or occipital lobe will create a homonymous hemianopia. The non-congruity of his visual field suggests optic tract or radiations.
- **Pituitary Adenoma or Lesion:** Although typically associated with bitemporal hemianopia due to compression of the optic chiasm, any expansion or unusual growth pattern could impact the visual pathway differently, especially if extending towards the optic tract.
- **Glaucoma:** Unlikely given his IOP and lack of typical optic disc changes, but always a consideration in visual field loss. However, his visual field defect pattern is classically suggestive of a central neurologic cause.
- **Retinal Pathology:** The bilaterality of his visual field defect and pattern is not consistent with an isolated retinal event or condition. His presenting symptoms were indeed suggestive to be purely ocular, however, on your exam it is quickly disproven.

Learning Points

- Recognize a homonymous hemianopia typically indicates a lesion along the post-chiasmal visual pathways, often involving the optic tract, radiations, or occipital lobe.
- Understand while pituitary lesions commonly cause bitemporal hemianopia, atypical presentations can occur if the lesion affects the optic tracts.
- Emphasize the importance of comprehensive neuroimaging to identify the precise location and source of visual field defects.
- Consider the potential for vascular events such as stroke in older patients presenting with sudden visual field loss and associated risk factors.

Questions

What are the potential neurologic implications of a right homonymous hemianopia?

A right homonymous hemianopia typically indicates a lesion in the left optic tract, lateral geniculate body, optic radiations, or occipital lobe. This pattern suggests post-chiasmal involvement, often pointing to a central neurologic pathology.

Why is further imaging essential in his evaluation?

Further imaging such as advanced MRI or CT angiography is essential to determine the exact location and nature of the lesion creating the visual field defect. It helps identify if the pituitary lesion is compressing the optic tract or if there is another underlying condition such as a vascular anomaly or an ischemic infarct, stroke.

How might a pituitary lesion affect the visual pathway differently than other intracranial pathologies?

A pituitary lesion typically compresses the optic chiasm leading to a bitemporal hemianopia. However, if the lesion grows atypically or is large enough, it may extend into the optic tract inducing a homonymous hemianopia. Other intracranial pathologies, such as stroke, more often directly affect the optic tract, radiations, or occipital lobe resulting in homonymous visual field defects.

What role does collaboration with neurology play in managing him?

Collaboration with neurology is crucial to accurately diagnose and manage the underlying cause of his visual field defect. Neurology will provide expertise in interpreting neuroimaging, identifying possible cerebral pathologies, and recommending an appropriate management plan.

Total Darkness

History of Present Illness (HPI)

A 74-year-old gentleman comes to see you after several months of intermittent episodes where his vision dims significantly, occasionally leading to complete bilateral blackouts lasting up to a minute. He's also experienced a couple recent instances of fainting. His last syncope event was associated severe hypotension, systolic in the 80s, requiring emergency medical attention at home and then a hospital admission. He tells you the hospital doctors were concerned about his "vagus nerve not working". He also asks you about specific effects and benefits of his newly prescribed medication, propranolol.

Review of Systems (ROS)

He describes vertiginous episodes when standing, transient dimming with sometimes complete vision loss, chest palpitations, as well as shortness of breath, all of which has increased in frequency over the previous two years.

Past Medical History (PMH)

He has a longstanding history of hypertension, hyperlipidemia, and type-2 diabetes, with challenges in managing these. However, his diabetes has been under better control with a recent A1C trending down at 7.1. Recently he was unable to complete a treadmill stress test due to blood pressure instability and tachycardia. He also has issues with sleep apnea and requires a CPAP overnight.

Family History (FH)

Both parents had type-2 diabetes, hypertension, and hyperlipidemia. His father had a stroke.

Medications and Allergies

He was recently prescribed propranolol. Lisinopril, metformin, atorvastatin, and nightly O2/CPAP. He has no known allergies to medications or environment.

Ophthalmic Examination

- **Best Corrected Visual Acuity (BCVA):** 20/30 OD, 20/40 OS.

- **Pupils:** Pupils equal, round, responsive to light and accommodation. No afferent pupillary defect. PERRLA, (-)APD.
- **Extraocular Muscles (EOMs):** Full, without diplopia.
- **Visual Field (VF):** Full OU.
- **Intraocular Pressure (IOP):** 15 mmHg OU.
- **Anterior Segment:** Clear cornea, deep and quiet anterior chamber, grade I nuclear and cortical lens changes OU.
- **Posterior Segment:** Optic nerve, macula, vitreous, unremarkable OU. Mild non-proliferative diabetic retinopathy without macular edema and early hypertensive arteriolosclerotic changes OU.
- **Optical Coherence Tomography (OCT):** OCT reveals mild rNFL thinning OU. Macula unremarkable without evidence of diabetic macular edema with good foveal contour OU.

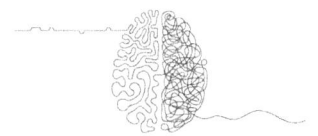

Think Deeper!

Discussion and Management

This gentleman with episodic bilateral loss of vision, hypotensive episodes, and syncope necessitates your broad diagnostic approach. Given his cardiovascular history, your primary concern is transient ischemia, possible autonomic dysfunction, with of course potential ocular complications. Your focus is on the interplay between his cardiovascular status and ocular symptoms, including the appropriateness of propranolol.

His documented hypotensive episode, coupled with visual disturbances and syncope, strongly suggest autonomic dysfunction. Specifically, vagus nerve dysregulation leading to unopposed sympathetic activity with subsequent cardiovascular and hemodynamic instability. Propranolol, a non-selective beta-blocker, is indicated to control his tachycardia but may unfortunately worsen his hypotension, potentially reducing cerebral perfusion and in fact facilitating his ocular symptoms. Addressing this possibility is crucial to maintain a balance of controlling his heart rate without exacerbating hypotensive events.

Transient ischemic attacks, or TIAs involve temporary disruptions in cerebral blood flow, leading to transient neurologic deficits including visual disturbances. His episodic loss of vision and syncope suggest cerebral hypoperfusion, warranting immediate neuroimaging via MRI and MRA looking for characteristic ischemic changes and/or vascular abnormalities. However, whether imaging is positive or negative, that does not solve the underlying source of his problems.

You therefore must address any uncontrolled cardiovascular risk factors, such as his hypertension, hyperlipidemia, and diabetes which of course increase the likelihood of vascular-related issues. An ECG and Echo (echocardiogram) is essential to evaluate cardiac function and detect potential sources or presence of emboli. Carotid duplex looking for significant carotid stenosis, which of course will also compromise cerebral perfusion with or without carotid atherosclerotic emboli. Continuous ambulatory monitoring via a Holter monitor may also be warranted to capture any spontaneous arrhythmic episodes which may have contributed to his previous events.

Postural orthostatic tachycardia syndrome (POTS) should be considered, characterized by hypotension and tachycardia upon standing, often leading to vertiginous symptoms like dizziness as well as visual disturbances and possible syncope. A tilt-table test can diagnose POTS by measuring heart rate and blood pressure responses to changes in posture.

Considering his diabetic and hypertensive retinopathy, rNFL compromise on OCT, his visual symptoms and ocular status is compounded by these chronic microvascular changes. He is particularly at high risk of developing normal tension glaucoma, NTG. Careful management of his diabetes and hypertension is of course very important from a purely ocular standpoint. Regular OCTs, visual fields, and retinal imaging will help you manage any progression of retinopathy and/or development of glaucoma. This will also allow you to properly recommend any adjustments in his overall medical management.

Your management involving neurology, cardiology, and endocrinology is imperative. Neurology will guide further investigations in terms of possible autonomic dysfunction, potentially linking POTS and TIA/stroke risk. Cardiology will optimize his cardiovascular management, addressing hypotension, arrhythmias, and potential embolic sources.

Endocrinology will help achieve tighter glycemic control and manage metabolic risk factors.

Differential Diagnoses and Medical Rationale

- **Transient Ischemic Attacks (TIAs):** Given the transient nature of his visual symptoms and syncope, TIAs are a primary concern. MRI and MRA are necessary to evaluate for ischemia or vascular abnormalities.
- **Autonomic Dysfunction/POTS/Orthostasis:** Potentially underlying his cardiovascular instability, contributing to episodes of syncope and visual disturbances.
- **Non-Arteritic Ischemic Optic Neuropathy (NAION):** Considered due to transient vision loss, though less likely without an acute persistent visual field deficit and/or decreased visual acuity.
- **Normal-Tension Glaucoma (NTG):** High-risk given his cardiovascular status and rNFL OCT findings, necessitating careful IOP monitoring, regular OCTs, and visual fields.

Learning Points

- Recognize the importance of considering transient ischemic attacks (TIAs) in individuals presenting with episodic vision loss, vertiginous symptoms, and/or syncope.
- Understand the role of autonomic dysfunction in contributing to cardiovascular instability and associated visual symptoms.

- Differentiate between vision loss due to vascular causes like acute NAION and chronic progressive conditions like normal-tension glaucoma.
- Highlight the necessity of comprehensive cardiovascular and neuroimaging assessments to identify potential central or vascular causes of transient vision loss.

Questions

How might autonomic dysfunction contribute to his symptoms?

Autonomic dysfunction can lead to cardiovascular instability, resulting in episodes of hypotension and syncope. This can reduce perfusion to critical ocular and cerebral structures, causing transient vision loss and other symptoms.

Why is family history significant in his case?

His family history is significant because it highlights a predisposition to cardiovascular diseases and type-2 diabetes, increasing his risk for vascular-related ophthalmopathy.

What are the key features of normal-tension glaucoma (NTG)?

Key features of NTG include progressive optic neuropathy with characteristic cupping, rNFL defect on OCT imaging, with or without visual field loss depending on severity, but with normal intraocular pressure. It is often associated with underlying vascular factors affecting optic nerve perfusion.

What role does propranolol play in his management, and what concerns does it raise?

Propranolol is prescribed to manage tachycardia presumed to arise from vagal nerve dysfunction or POTS. However, it raises concerns due to his acute hypotensive episodes, for which propranolol may only exacerbate his visual symptoms and ocular status by reducing perfusion to critical ocular and cerebral structures.

What is the importance of neuroimaging in his evaluation?

Neuroimaging is crucial to explore potential central causes of his symptoms, such as transient ischemic attacks or other forms of vascular compromise to the eye and visual pathway. It will also help identify any structural abnormalities which may be contributing to his visual and overall symptoms.

Skewed Perspectives

History of Present Illness (HPI)

A 35-year-old gentleman is in your chair noticing sudden-onset and persistent oblique diplopia that began a few weeks ago. He believes it has been progressively worsening and is most noticeable when looking upwards or to his right.

Review of Systems (ROS)

Over the past few months he has been having intermittent headaches which are mostly localized to his forehead and around his eyes, which tend to be more pronounced in the mornings. He tells you about transient visual obscurations or auras which seem to occur around the time of his headaches. He has not had any nausea or vomiting. He also reluctantly mentions he must be getting old since turning 30 and thinks he is "forgetting things".

Past Medical History (PMH)

He has been generally healthy with no chronic illnesses or significant medical issues in the past.

Family History (FH)

Maternal uncle who underwent surgery for a benign "brain tumor" in his late forties. Both parents healthy without medical issues.

Medications and Allergies

He takes no prescription medications and has no known allergies to medications or environmental issues.

Ophthalmic Examination

- **Best Corrected Visual Acuity (BCVA):** OD 20/25, OS 20/20.
- **Pupils:** Anisocoria, OD>OS, OD>>>OS in bright illumination.
- **Extraocular Muscles (EOMs):** Restriction in upward gaze and reduction of depression in right gaze OD, with diplopia.
- **Visual Field (VF):** Enlarged blind spot OD. Full with normal blind spot OS.
- **Intraocular Pressure (IOP):** 21 OD, 16 OS
- **Anterior Segment:** Clear cornea, deep and quiet anterior chamber, clear lens OU.
- **Posterior Segment:** Bilateral disc edema, more pronounced OD. Macula, vessels, vitreous, retina

unremarkable OU.

- **Optical Coherence Tomography (OCT):** OCT shows subtle retinal nerve fiber layer thickening OD. Normal optic nerve OS. Macula clear with good foveal contour OU.

Neurologic Examination

- **Cranial Nerves:** No additional cranial nerve abnormalities on exam.
- **Motor and Sensory Function:** Normal strength and sensation throughout.

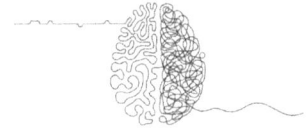

Think Deeper!

Discussion and Management

Given his symptoms of diplopia, papilledema, restricted movement of his right eye, and your OCT findings confirming the presence of disc edema, you highly suspect an active and ongoing retrobulbar and/or intracranial process. You urgently order an MRI brain with and without contrast which unfortunately reveals a lesion within the cavernous sinus. Although biopsies within the cavernous sinus are not always indicated or feasibly safe, this gentleman requires it. Histology shows psammomatous characteristics with multiple concentrically laminated calcium concretions, confirming a classic diagnosis of cavernous sinus meningioma.

The cavernous sinus is a venous plexus located on either side of the pituitary gland. It contains important structures such as the internal carotid artery and cranial nerves III, IV, V (V1 and V2), and VI. Compression or displacement of these structures can lead to symptoms like progressive diplopia, ischemic vision loss, and even alterations in facial sensation and function.

Meningiomas are non-malignant benign masses which arise from the meninges, specifically from the meningothelial (arachnoid cap) cells. They are most common in middle-aged adults and tend to grow slowly, sometimes developing within the cavernous sinus or extending into the cavernous sinus from adjacent areas. Cavernous sinus meningiomas can produce a variety of very predictable signs and symptoms when you first understand the relationship of anatomic structure and function within this space. In this gentleman's case, a right IVn palsy is apparent and perhaps early IIIn involvement with a sluggish or non-responsive mydriatic pupil OD.

You consider some of the many predictable possibilities...

- IIIn, IVn, VIn palsies creating corresponding strabismus and resultant diplopia.
- Facial pain or paresthesia involving the V1 or V2 distribution of the trigeminal nerve.
- Proptosis (exophthalmos) secondary to increasing intracranial pressure can occur.

- Ptosis as a result of full or partial IIIn palsy with or without anisocoria, a mydriatic pupil, depending on if the parasympathetic fibers which run alongside the path of the IIIn are being impinged upon.
- Loss of vision or visual field defects, understanding the internal carotid artery (ICA) which supply's the ophthalmic artery can pose risk of ischemic optic neuropathy, if compressive obstruction ensues or thromboembolic events occur.
- Progressive and refractory headache.

Management strategies will of course involve a team approach. Surgical resection is the preferred treatment when feasible, aiming to remove the mass while preserving neurologic function. The decision for surgery is guided by factors such as its size, exact location, growth rate, symptoms, as well as his overall medical history. Given its complex location, you know attempting a partial or complete resection will pose significant risks.

For residual or recurrent meningiomas, especially in anatomically challenging locations like the cavernous sinus, radiotherapy including stereotactic techniques like gamma-knife or cyber-knife provides targeted treatment options that minimize damage to surrounding tissues. These methods are highly effective for controlling growth and reducing symptoms over time. Additionally, pharmacological management primarily utilizing corticosteroids can help reduce peritumoral edema and help alleviate signs and symptoms rather quickly.

Your understanding the chronic nature of meningiomas and potential for recurrence, long-term surveillance and management is essential. Regular follow-up with neuroimaging is critical to manage stability or progression, and adjustments to his treatment plan may be necessary based on future findings. Post surgical resolution of his cranial nerve palsy and disc edema is possible, however, you must prepare him for the possibility of permanent deficits. This includes persistent diplopia, which can be managed with prism correction or possibly future strabismus surgery. Because of potential optic atrophy, he also needs to be aware of the possibility of a permanent reduction in acuity and/or visual field deficit.

Differential Diagnoses and Medical Rationale

- **Meningioma:** Primary diagnosis supported by imaging and histological findings.
- **Pituitary Adenoma:** Considered for its potential to cause similar symptoms, however, a pituitary adenoma increasing intracranial pressure to the point of disc edema and an isolated IVn palsy is extraordinarily unlikely. The lack of endocrine signs and/or symptoms also points away from a pituitary source.
- **Craniopharyngioma:** The presence of calcification might suggest this diagnosis, but it also usually presents with significant endocrine symptoms.
- **Schwannoma:** Although cranial nerve involvement possibly suggests this type of mass, the histological features observed are characteristic of meningioma.

Learning Points

- Recognize the characteristic presentation of meningiomas, including symptoms such as diplopia, headaches, and papilledema.
- Understand the importance of MRI and histological analysis in diagnosing meningiomas and differentiating them from other intracranial masses.
- Understand the role and risks of surgical resection in the management of meningiomas and the factors influencing surgical decisions.
- Highlight the use of radiotherapy techniques like gamma-knife or cyber-knife for residual or recurrent meningiomas, particularly in challenging locations.

Questions

What imaging modality is crucial for diagnosing meningiomas and why?

MRI is crucial for diagnosing meningiomas as it provides detailed images of the brain and can identify the location, size, and effect of the mass on adjacent structures. Histological analysis further confirms the diagnosis.

What are the potential complications of meningiomas located in the cavernous sinus?

Complications include cranial nerve compression leading to diplopia, vision loss, alterations in facial sensation, and potentially other neurologic deficits depending on the extent of growth.

How does radiotherapy help in managing residual or recurrent meningiomas?

Radiotherapy, including stereotactic techniques like gamma-knife or cyber-knife, targets the mass precisely, minimizing damage to surrounding tissues and effectively controlling growth and reducing symptoms.

What role do corticosteroids play in the management of meningiomas?

Corticosteroids help reduce peritumoral inflammation and edema, alleviating symptoms quickly and improving neurologic function while definitive treatments like surgery or radiotherapy are being planned.

Why is long-term surveillance important in patients with meningiomas?

Long-term surveillance is important to monitor for stability or progression, detect recurrence early, and adjust the treatment plan as necessary.

Driver Can't Drive

History of Present Illness (HPI)

A 60-year-old gentleman urgently comes to see you. He is a truck driver who suddenly noticed he "can't see" when waking up that morning. He describes it as a "shadow" blocking half of his vision. He has no vision or medical insurance.

Review of Systems (ROS)

He reports no pain, headaches, numbness, movement, or

speech difficulties. He occasionally experiences "light-headedness". Generally, he feels fatigued quite often.

Past Medical History (PMH)

He has a history of hypertension, which has been managed sporadically due to lack of medical insurance. There is also suspicion of hyperlipidemia, which has never been formally diagnosed or treated. He has a 30 pack-year history of smoking.

Family History (FH)

He has a family history of cardiovascular disease; both parents had hypertension and his father had a stroke in his late sixties.

Medications and Allergies

He takes no medication other than OTC "caffeine pills" to help him stay awake while driving. He has no known medication or environmental allergies.

Ophthalmic Examination

- **Best Corrected Visual Acuity (BCVA)**: 20/30 OD, 20/40 OS.
- **Pupils**: Pupils equal, round, reactive to light and accommodation, no afferent pupillary defect. PERRLA, (-)APD.
- **Extraocular Muscles (EOMs)**: Full, without diplopia.
- **Visual Field (VF)**: Congruous left homonymous hemianopia.
- **Intraocular Pressure (IOP)**: 21 OD, 20 OS.

- **Anterior Segment**: Clear cornea, deep and quiet anterior chamber, early nuclear and cortical lens changes OU.
- **Posterior Segment**: Optic disc, macula, vessels, vitreous, retina unremarkable OU. No evidence of disc edema or retinopathy OU.
- **Optical Coherence Tomography (OCT)**: Normal optic nerve and retinal nerve fiber layer (rNFL) OU, macula clear with good foveal contour OU.

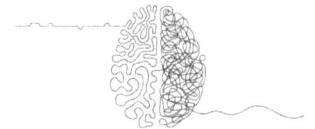

Think Deeper!

Discussion and Management

His presentation with a sudden congruous left homonymous hemianopia of course raises your immediate concern, specifically in terms of an acute cerebrovascular event or stroke affecting his right occipital lobe or in the vicinity of the right parieto-occipital region. His sudden onset of symptoms, particularly without preceding trauma or other visual disturbances, points you towards an emergent ischemic stroke rather than a more slowly occurring hemorrhagic event.

Understanding the urgency of timely treatment in the event of an acute ischemic stroke, you immediately send him to an emergency department, a stroke center equipped for immediate imaging and possible treatment. A non-contrast head CT is standard protocol done immediately on arrival and is critical in confirming your suspicion, but also rules out possible causes such as a hemorrhagic or aneurysmal stroke, complications from an unknown mass, and others. Non-contrast CT is fast and easy and most necessary to exclude hemorrhagic stroke for which the management will be far different.

In terms of ischemic stroke, if confirmed and he is within the therapeutic window from symptom onset, intravenous tissue plasminogen activator (tPA) may be administered. TPA can initiate a biochemical breakdown of an occlusive thrombus, improve perfusion to the ischemic cerebral region, significantly improving his outcome if administered promptly. However, the risks and benefits must be carefully weighed, particularly given his hypertension and smoking history which may predispose him to hemorrhagic complications. In the event a hemorrhagic stroke is discovered, tPA is of course an absolute contraindication.

You are reminded of the importance to understand the action of tissue plasminogen activator (tPA). It is a protein involved in the breakdown of thrombi, or fibrinolysis. It is particularly effective in dissolving thrombi that form in blood vessels, not only as a thrombolytic agent in the treatment of acute ischemic stroke but also in myocardial infarction and pulmonary embolism. This occurs over several steps...

1. *Activation of Plasminogen*: tPA converts plasminogen, an inactive precursor, into plasmin, an active enzyme. Plasminogen is naturally present in blood and tissues and gets incorporated into the clot as it forms.

2. *Binding to Fibrin*: tPA has a high affinity with fibrin, the primary protein that makes up blood clots. It binds to the fibrin within the thrombus, where it efficiently activates the conversion of plasminogen to plasmin.

3. *Plasminogen to Plasmin Conversion*: Once bound to fibrin, tPA catalyzes the conversion of plasminogen to plasmin. This reaction happens more efficiently on the surface of fibrin than in the circulating blood, which helps to localize the activity of plasmin to the site of the clot.

4. *Degradation of Fibrin*: Plasmin is a powerful enzyme that degrades fibrin into smaller fragments. This breakdown of fibrin dissolves the structural foundation of the thrombus, leading to the disintegration of the clot.

5. *Restoration of Blood Flow*: As the clot dissolves, blood flow is restored through the previously obstructed vessel, which helps to alleviate the symptoms and reduce the risk of damage due to the blockage.

The effectiveness of tPA is highly dependent on the timing of administration. For instance, in the case of ischemic stroke it is most effective when administered within 3-4.5 hours from the onset of symptoms.

Following any acute management he receives, long-term strategies need to be put in place to reduce his risk of recurrent stroke. These include strict blood pressure control, initiation of statin therapy to manage his hyperlipidemia, and smoking cessation. Anti-platelet therapy such as aspirin or clopidogrel may also be recommended to help prevent further thrombotic events. Given his socioeconomic status and lack of medical insurance, it will be very important to connect him with community health resources or social services that can provide ongoing support including his inability to drive for a living.

Differential Diagnoses and Rationale

- **Ischemic Stroke**: Primary consideration given his pattern of visual loss and sudden onset. Immediate imaging and neurologic evaluation can confirm the presence of an infarct.
- **Hemorrhagic Stroke:** CT must be performed immediately and will either exclude or confirm this possibility.
- **Compressive Lesion or Mass Effect**: Less likely due to the acute onset without progressive symptoms. CT will exclude this possibility.
- **Migraine with Aura**: Considered due to his visual symptoms, but less likely given the persistence of his vision loss, his age, and lack of headache.

Learning Points

- Recognize the importance of rapid assessment and intervention in individuals presenting with acute visual changes suggestive of stroke.
- Understand the need for comprehensive imaging to differentiate between ischemic and hemorrhagic stroke and to rule out other potential causes such as mass effects.
- Emphasize the significance of addressing modifiable risk factors, including hypertension, hyperlipidemia,

and smoking to prevent recurrent cerebrovascular events.

- Appreciate the socioeconomic factors that can impact access to healthcare and the importance of connecting people with community resources for ongoing support.

Questions

What are key imaging modalities used to diagnose an ischemic stroke?

Imaging modalities include MRI with and without contrast of the brain, focusing on cerebral vasculature. However, urgent non-contrast CT is faster, easier, more accessible, and most appropriate to immediately rule-out a hemorrhagic stroke.

Why is immediate referral to an emergency department critical in his case?

It is to rapidly assess and manage a potential ischemic stroke, reducing risk of further neurologic damage and improving outcomes with timely tPA intervention.

How does the administration of tPA help in the management of ischemic stroke?

TPA helps dissolve the thrombus and restore perfusion to the affected area of the brain, significantly improving outcomes if administered within the therapeutic window from symptom onset.

What long-term management strategies are essential for stroke prevention in for him?

Strategies include strict blood pressure control, statin therapy, smoking cessation, anti-platelet therapy, lifestyle changes, and regular follow-up to manage and reduce his risk factors.

What are potential complications of administering tPA and how should they be monitored?

Potential complications include bleeding, particularly hemorrhagic transformation of an ischemic stroke. Individuals need to be closely managed for signs of worsening neurologic status and bleeding complications after administration.

Little Girl Seeing Rainbows

History of Present Illness (HPI)

A young mom brings her 6-year-old little girl to see you. She was sent home from school due to experiencing visual disturbances she describes as seeing "rainbows". She tells you the rainbows are still there while sitting on her mom's lap in your chair. It may not be the first time, as her mom recalls her talking about "rainbows" in the past.

Review of Systems (ROS)

She has experienced this sensation more than once, and more often when playing outside or when she's had a bad day at school. It can persist for just a few minutes or occasionally for a couple of hours. Her mom has not noticed any unusual behavior before, during, or after these episodes, and your little patient has not had any pain or headache.

Past Medical History (PMH)

She was born with a ventricular septal defect (VSD) which resolved without surgical intervention. She's had previous issues with possible dehydration and was seen by her pediatrician for a couple episodes of near syncope when playing outside.

Family History (FH)

Mother with migraine history. No neurologic disorders or genetic disease.

Medications and Allergies

No medications. She has no known allergies to medications, food, or environmental factors.

Ophthalmic Examination

- **Best Corrected Visual Acuity (BCVA):** 20/20 OU.
- **Pupils:** Pupils equal, round, responsive to light and accommodation, no afferent pupillary defect. PERRLA, (-)APD.
- **Extraocular Muscles (EOMs):** Full, no diplopia.
- **Visual Field (VF):** Confrontation, full OU.
- **Intraocular Pressure (IOP):** 15mmHg OU.
- **Anterior Segment:** Clear cornea, deep and quiet anterior chamber, clear lens OU.
- **Posterior Segment:** Optic disc, macula, vessels, vitreous, retina unremarkable.
- **Optical Coherence Tomography (OCT):** Not performed.

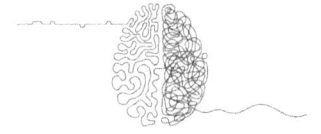

Think Deeper!

Discussion and Management

This little one's clinical scenario of intermittent and transient scintillating scotoma is indicative of several potential underlying conditions, ranging from neurologic to cardiovascular. Considering her mom's history of migraine, your initial thought is early onset of ocular migraine with aura despite her young age. Migraines in children, though rare, can manifest with visual auras without the subsequent headache phase. These auras often involve scintillating scotomas and can be triggered by factors such as dietary issues, physical exertion, and/or stress.

In terms of nutritional factors, migraine in children has been linked to certain vitamin and mineral deficiencies. One key deficiency is in vitamin D, where low levels have been associated with increased frequency and severity of migraines. Vitamin D is crucial for overall neurologic function, and its anti-inflammatory properties may play a significant role in preventing migraines.

Another important vitamin is riboflavin, or vitamin B2. Deficiency in riboflavin is connected to migraines due to its role in mitochondrial energy production. When riboflavin levels are low, mitochondrial dysfunction can occur which is believed to be a factor in the development of migraines.

Folate, known as vitamin B9 is also essential. A deficiency in folate can be associated with migraines, particularly in individuals with certain genetic variations affecting folate metabolism. Adequate levels of folate are necessary for proper neurotransmitter synthesis and function.

Vitamin B12 is another vital nutrient linked to migraines. Deficiency in B12 can lead to various neurologic symptoms including migraines, as it is essential for neuronal integrity and hematopoiesis.

Although not a vitamin, magnesium is a mineral which plays a significant role in the context of migraines. Magnesium deficiency is commonly linked to migraines because it is involved in numerous cellular processes, including nerve function and the regulation of vascular tone.

Because of her age, you also consider the possibility of seizure activity which can be associated with migraine in children, preceding with scintillating type "rainbow" auras. This relationship is found in a condition known as migralepsy, where the visual aura is closely followed by a seizure disturbance. The connection between migraine and seizure disorders can be explained by overlapping pathophysiological mechanisms, including shared genetic factors, alterations in brain excitability, and similar triggers such as stress, sleep disturbances, and hormonal imbalance.

Childhood seizure disturbances can be "silent" or manifest as "absence" seizures. Absence seizures, also known as petit-mal seizures, are characterized by brief sudden lapses in attention and consciousness without the convulsive activity typically associated with other types of seizures. These seizures are not uncommon in children and can last for just a few seconds, often going unnoticed or being mistaken for daydreaming.

Given her history of VSD, your most important next step is to first rule out any residual or related cardiovascular source. Although her VSD reportedly resolved per mom without surgical intervention, her current status cannot be assumed. This history alone suggests her potential predisposition to continuing cardiovascular dysfunction or hemodynamic instability. The manifestation of visual symptoms due to transient cerebral ischemia during periods of increased physical activity is a real possibility.

Finally, her episodes during or following playing outside raise the possibility of hypoglycemia and/or dehydration, both of which can induce transient visual symptoms in children. Again, a review of her diet as well as hydration during physical activities is very important.

You coordinate to re-evaluate her cardiac status with pediatric cardiology, and again, this your top priority. If she is cleared, studies such as EEG, MRI brain, labs for glucose, electrolytes, and nutritional screenings can be pursued to ensure a thorough investigation.

Differential Diagnoses and Rationale

- **Early Onset Ocular Migraine:** High likelihood given her symptomatology and familial predisposition. Migraines in children can present with visual auras without subsequent headaches.

- **Congenital Cardiac VSD Status:** Due to her past medical history, with symptoms potentially linked to transient ischemic episodes. Residual cardiovascular issues from her VSD could lead to circulatory insufficiency or hemodynamic instability.
- **Seizure Disorder:** To be considered if other sources are ruled out. Visual auras associated with absence seizures is plausible.
- **Nutritional Deficiencies:** Deficiencies in Vitamin D, B2 (riboflavin), magnesium, and others have been linked to increased migraine susceptibility in children.
- **Hypoglycemia and/or Dehydration:** Not uncommon in active children, especially if episodes correlate with physical exertion combined with a questionable diet and insufficient hydration.

Learning Points

- Understand the pathophysiology of ocular migraines, including the role of cortical spreading depression and the neurovascular mechanisms involved in the aura phase.
- Know that absence seizures can be associated and follow migrainous visual auras in children.
- Recognize the potential impact of congenital cardiac conditions on cerebral perfusion and the importance of ruling out residual cardiovascular concerns.
- Emphasize the need for a comprehensive approach to managing pediatric patients with visual disturbances, including neurologic, cardiovascular, and nutritional evaluations.

- Appreciate the importance of educating families on maintaining adequate hydration and balanced nutrition to prevent and manage triggers.

Questions

What are some key mechanisms involved in the pathophysiology of ocular migraine and seizure disorders in children?

The connection between migraines and seizures can be explained by overlapping pathophysiological mechanisms, including shared genetic factors, alterations in brain excitability, and similar triggers such as stress, sleep disturbances, and hormonal changes.

How can congenital cardiac conditions contribute to visual disturbances in children?

Congenital cardiac conditions can predispose children to circulatory insufficiency or hemodynamic instability, leading to transient cerebral ischemia during periods of increased physical activity which can manifest as visual disturbances.

What are some differential diagnoses for children presenting with visual disturbances, and how are they distinguished?

Differential diagnoses include early onset ocular migraine, congenital cardiac conditions, seizure disorders, nutritional deficiencies, hypoglycemia, and dehydration. They can be distinguished by clinical presentation, associated symptoms, and diagnostic investigations such as MRI, EEG, ECG, labs, and nutritional screenings.

What role does educating families on maintaining adequate hydration and balanced nutrition play in managing children with visual disturbances?

Educating families on maintaining adequate hydration and balanced nutrition helps prevent and manage possible triggers, reducing risk of associated issues such as hypoglycemia and dehydration.

***

Strange Sensations

History of Present Illness (HPI)

A 47-year-old lady is in your chair. Recently she has been experiencing an unusual sensation in vision on her right side which she can't seem to describe. It is episodic lasting anywhere from a few minutes to a few hours, and occurs sporadically throughout the day without any clear trigger.

Review of Systems (ROS)

She describes transient vertiginous symptoms and unsteady gait, particularly during the visual episodes. She denies any recent fever, weight loss, or night sweats, but mentions occasional mild headaches when the episodes occur.

Past Medical History (PMH)

She has been experiencing migraine headaches for nearly 10 years, characterized by unilateral throbbing pain, photophobia, and nausea with occasional scintillating scotomas. She has a history of hypertension and a recent diagnosis of hyperlipidemia. She had an intracranial meningioma resected 5 years ago, with no recurrence noted on follow-up imaging.

Family History (FH)

Mother and father with hypertension and hyperlipidemia. Father had a stroke in his 50's.

Medications and Allergies

Amlodipine 5 mg, atorvastatin 10 mg daily, acetaminophen as needed and a daily multivitamin.

Ophthalmic Examination

- **Best Corrected Visual Acuity (BCVA):** 20/20 OU.
- **Pupils:** Pupils equal, round, reactive to light and accommodation, no afferent pupillary defect. PERRLA, (-)APD.
- **Extraocular Muscles (EOMs):** Full, without diplopia.
- **Visual Field (VF):** Full OU.
- **Intraocular Pressure (IOP):** 19 OD, 20 OS.
- **Anterior Segment:** Clear cornea, deep and quiet anterior chamber, clear lens OU.
- **Posterior Segment:** Optic nerve, macula, vessels, vitreous, retina unremarkable OU. No evidence of disc edema OU.
- **Optical Coherence Tomography (OCT):** Normal optic nerve and retinal nerve fiber layer (rNFL) with no disc edema OU. Macula clear with good foveal contour OU.

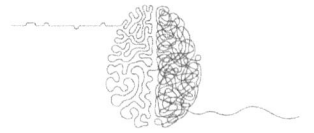

Think Deeper!

Discussion and Management

She comes to you with a complex scenario, including non-specific transient visual obscurations and accompanying neurologic symptoms. Of course, you immediately have concerns far beyond ocular migraines. Her history of hypertension, hyperlipidemia, and previous meningioma resection creates layers of possible differential diagnoses.

Considering the episodic nature of her visual disturbances combined with vertiginous symptoms, unsteady gait, and mild headaches, suggests to you the possibility of transient ischemia. Understanding her hypertension and hyperlipidemia increases this risk for transient cerebrovascular events, you immediately order MRA and MRI of the brain with contrast, looking for any acute evidence of ischemia, micro-infarcts, or vascular abnormalities.

You also order and obtain a carotid duplex, assessing for significant carotid artery stenosis which can contribute to possible transient ischemia. Additionally, an ECG, Holter monitor, and echocardiogram can help identify a cardiac source for her symptoms. This includes various arrhythmia's and/or valvular disease increasing risk of thrombotic or atherosclerotic emboli.

Her possible transient ischemic "attacks", TIA's, are brief episodes of neurologic dysfunction caused by temporary disruption of blood perfusion to areas of the brain, spinal cord, and/or retina. These episodes usually last for a short period, often resolving within minutes to hours and do not normally create permanent neurologic deficits. The pathophysiology involves temporary vascular occlusion of key vessels as a result of atherosclerotic plaque formation, thereby narrowing vessels and reducing perfusion. These plaques can also rupture leading to associated thrombus formation.

An additional source of TIAs are thrombotic or atherosclerotic emboli originating elsewhere such as the heart, traveling and finding their way to the cerebral vasculature resulting in temporary occlusion. Arrhythmia's like atrial fibrillation are not uncommon and contribute to this risk by promoting stasis and subsequent thrombogenesis within the cardiac chambers, with thrombi being shot out into systemic circulation. Valvular disease and the release of atheroemboli is another common mechanism of upstream vascular occlusion.

The pathophysiology of TIAs can be intricately linked to both hypo-coagulable and hyper-coagulable states, each influencing cerebrovascular perfusion through distinct mechanisms. Hypercoagulability is characterized by an enhanced propensity for thrombus formation within the systemic vasculature, predisposing individuals to thromboembolic events. Genetic predispositions, such as Factor V Leiden mutation or the prothrombin G20210A mutation, will increase coagulative risk and therefore potential cerebral thromboemboli. Additionally, chronic hypercoagulable states can induce endothelial damage and vascular fragility, also contributing to potential cerebrovascular insults.

Conversely, hypocoagulability is a deficiency in the blood's capacity to maintain "protective clotting", thereby predisposing to hemorrhagic events. While less commonly associated with the etiology of TIAs, hypocoagulability can indirectly precipitate cerebrovascular instability. Hemorrhages resulting from inadequate hemostasis can lead to secondary vasospasm or intracranial pressure induced ischemia, thereby mimicking the clinical presentation of occlusive TIAs.

The delicate equilibrium of hemostatic mechanisms is key in mitigating the risk of TIAs. Hypercoagulable states primarily augment the risk through thromboembolic phenomena, while hypocoagulable states can also compromise cerebrovascular integrity through hemorrhagic events.

Sometimes, spontaneous cerebral vasospasm can occur constricting and reducing perfusion temporarily. Vasospasm can be influenced by various factors, including fluctuations in blood pressure and certain medications. Additionally, the cerebral microvasculature can be compromised by chronic conditions such as hypertension and diabetes, leading to narrowing and temporary occlusion in the case of TIA's.

You consider her very significant history of meningioma resection. Although previous follow-up imaging showed no recurrence, you realize residual or a new occurrence producing intermittent compression is always possible. Your pending imaging order will also assess this and look for other intracranial pathology.

Early demyelinating optic neuritis or other inflammatory etiologies affecting the optic nerve can present in similar fashion. While her OCT findings are normal, it is important to consider other diagnostic tools such as visual evoked potentials (VEP) to evaluate functional integrity of the optic nerve and visual pathway, if other diagnostics prove to be inconclusive.

You know management must involve addressing the underlying source. With respect to likely TIAs, controlling cardiovascular risk factors such as arrhythmia, hypertension, hyperlipidemia, and others through medication, diet, and lifestyle is most important. Anti-platelet therapy such as aspirin and/or clopidogrel if indicated will reduce the risk of further ischemic events or stroke. For any identified recurrent or newly discovered meningioma, surgical or radiotherapy options may be considered depending on its extent and location.

Differential Diagnoses and Rationale

- **Transient Ischemic Attack (TIA):** The episodic nature of her symptoms and risk factors such as hypertension and hyperlipidemia make TIA a primary consideration. MRI and MRA are necessary to evaluate for ischemia or vascular abnormalities.
- **Recurrent or New Meningioma:** A residual recurrence or new occurrence creating compression and/or varying intracranial pressure, with transient right-sided visual field obscurations. Repeat neuroimaging is warranted.
- **Migraine with Aura:** Although her history includes migraine with aura, the variability of episodes with

additional neurologic symptoms like ataxia warrant further investigation beyond migraine.

- **Retinal Migraine:** Rare but possible, especially if associated with a history of migraines. A detailed retinal examination and fluorescein angiography may be warranted.
- **Occipital Lobe:** Occipital lobe pathology can induce visual disturbances. MRI of the brain with contrast is necessary to identify any mass effect or structural abnormalities.
- **Optic Neuritis:** Inflammation of the optic nerve can cause transient visual loss, however, the episodic nature of her symptoms points away from it. MRI and visual evoked potentials (VEP) can provide pertinent diagnostic information if indicated.
- **Giant Cell Arteritis/Temporal Arteritis:** Less common in her age group, but GCA can trigger significant visual symptoms. ESR and CRP levels, along with a temporal artery biopsy if indicated can further assess the possibility.

Learning Points:

- Recognize the clinical features of ocular migraine, including transient visual disturbances with or without headache, and differentiate it from more ominous conditions such as transient ischemic attacks (TIAs) or occipital lobe pathology.
- Understand the role of MRI and MRA in evaluating patients with unusual visual symptoms to rule out urgent conditions such acute infarction, expanding mass, or other structural abnormalities. Early and

accurate imaging is crucial for appropriate diagnosis and management.

- Evaluate the significance of cardiovascular risk factors such as arrhythmias, coagulopathies, hypertension, and hyperlipidemia in individuals presenting with visual disturbances. These risk factors increase the likelihood of transient ischemic cerebrovascular events, TIAs.

Questions

What are her key risk factors for transient ischemic attacks (TIAs)?

In her case, this includes hypertension, hyperlipidemia, and history of migraines. These conditions increase risk of cerebrovascular events.

How can MRI and MRA help in diagnosing the underlying cause of her symptoms?

They can help identify signs of ischemia, vascular abnormalities, or structural lesions in the brain that can be the source of her visual disturbances and neurologic symptoms.

Why is it important to consider her history of meningioma resection in evaluating her current symptoms?

It is important because risk of residual recurrent meningioma, or a newly formed meningioma, can directly compress areas along the visual pathway or other neurologic structures leading to her current symptoms. Increasing intracranial pressure (ICP) can also be a source of her symptoms.

What role do visual evoked potentials (VEP) play in diagnosing optic neuritis?

Visual evoked potentials (VEP) measure the electrical activity in the occipital cortex in response to visual stimuli, helping evaluate the functional integrity of the optic nerve and pathway. It can be utilized in her case to support or refute a diagnosis of optic neuritis.

Boxcars

History of Present Illness (HPI)

An 81-year-old gentleman is in your chair with a sudden onset of double vision he describes as "boxcars" when looking at lights. He first noticed this one morning several weeks ago when waking up, and it has not gone away. In fact, the "boxcars" seem to move further apart as the day goes on and it is impossible for him to read or drive. He tells you it gets better if he keeps one eye closed, which is how he has been walking around. He also mentions mild intermittent headaches which he has not had before.

Review of Systems (ROS)

For many years, he has experienced what he believes is vertigo. He has had some weight loss over the last couple years. He has no nausea, vomiting, fever, chills, night sweats, or recent illnesses. He has occasional numbness and tingling in his feet.

Past Medical History (PMH)

He was recently diagnosed with type-2 diabetes just a couple years ago. He has longstanding hypertension, hyperlipidemia, and recently diabetic neuropathy in his lower extremities. He did have a minor myocardial infarction (MI) last year which did not require anything other than medical managment. No associated stroke or stroke history. He had previous cataract surgery in each eye.

Family History (FH)

His father had a history of stroke and hypertension. His mother had type-2 diabetes with diabetic retinopathy. He remembers her having one of the first "laser treatments" available in the U.S.

Medications & Allergies

Daily Metformin 1000 mg, Lisinopril 20 mg, atorvastatin 40 mg, gabapentin 300 mg, aspirin 81 mg, metoprolol 50 mg. He has no known allergies to medications, foods, or environmental factors.

Ophthalmic Examination:

- **Best Corrected Visual Acuity (BCVA):** 20/30 OD, 20/40 OS.
- **Pupils:** Pupils equal, round, reactive to light and accommodation, no afferent pupillary defect. PERRLA, (-)APD.
- **Extraocular Muscles (EOMs):** Limited abduction of the right eye with diplopia on right gaze.
- **Visual Field (VF):** Non-congruous left homonymous hemianopic visual field defect.
- **Intraocular Pressure (IOP):** 14 OD, 12 OS.

- **Anterior Segment:** Cornea with mild anterior basement membrane dystrophy (ABMD), deep and quiet anterior chamber, pseudophakia with posterior chamber intra-ocular lens (PC IOL) OU.
- **Posterior Segment:** Optic nerve, vessels, vitreous, retina unremarkable OU. No evidence of disc edema OU. Macula with slight RPE mottling and drusen OU.
- **Optical Coherence Tomography (OCT):** Normal optic nerve and retinal nerve fiber layer (rNFL) OU. Macula with RPE changes, drusen, and small drusenoid RPE detachments without subretinal fluid (SRF) OU.

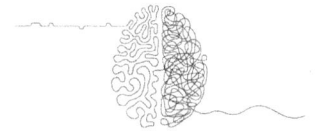

Think Deeper!

Discussion and Management

This gentleman will prove to be your forever reminder of the importance to never assume a diagnosis based on initial impressions. This is particularly true with individuals having complex medical histories.

In his case, it was easy for you to fall into the trap of assuming an elderly individual with diabetes and acute diplopia developed a typical diabetic VI nerve palsy. However, you thought twice, because you learned a long time ago to assume nothing and now know the importance of exploring all possible sources.

His classic VIn palsy and horizontal diplopia does strongly suggest microvascular neuropathy. Microvascular ischemia is a well-known cause of isolated cranial nerve palsies in diabetes, particularly involving the III, IV, and VI cranial nerves, with the VIn most commonly affected. These palsies typically present with sudden-onset diplopia without pain, and are often self-limiting resolving over weeks to months. However, his recent headaches as well as his age prompts you to investigate further.

Your decision to order neuroimaging is absolutely necessary and indicated. MRI with and without contrast is the imaging modality of choice for identifying structural lesions such as a mass, aneurysm, or other intracranial pathology which could compress or impinge upon the cranial nerves. MRI with FIESTA protocol is especially appropriate in his case, as it is a targeted advanced technique looking specifically for potential cranial nerve pathology.

His MRI shockingly revealed a pituitary lesion with suprasellar extension, impinging and compressing the right optic tract and VIn, creating his clinical picture and resultant horizontal diplopia.

Pituitary adenomas are the most common type of pituitary lesions and can induce a wide range of signs and symptoms, depending on their size and hormones they may secrete. Prolactinomas are the most common of the pituitary adenomas. Rarely an adenoma may expand and increase in size to extend beyond the sella turcica and may not compress the optic chiasm producing a bitemporal hemianopia, but instead primarily affect the optic tract leading to a left or right hemianopic visual field defect. The VI nerve is also particularly susceptible to compression due to its long intracranial course and proximity to the sella turcica, traveling within the cavernous sinus.

It is always vital to maintain a high index of suspicion for alternative diagnoses and to consider a broad differential diagnosis, again to assume nothing. This includes not only diabetic cranial nerve neuropathy but also neoplastic and compressive lesions, vascular anomalies, and other intracranial pathologies.

Pituitary adenomas are typically managed with surgical resection, particularly if they are producing signs and symptoms or are hormonally active. Aside from visual field deficits, hyperprolactinemia, growth hormone (GH) excess, Cushing's disease via increased adrenocorticotropic hormone (ACTH) secretion, other excessive activity can occur depending on the type of adenoma. Conversely, these may be diminished if purely mass effect and compression compromise normal pituitary function and secretion.

In his particular scenario, neurosurgery consult is absolutely necessary. Transsphenoidal surgery is the standard approach for resecting pituitary adenomas, as it allows direct access to the sella turcica with minimal disruption to surrounding structures. Of course, future endocrinology evaluations will always be necessary to assess pituitary function and manage potential hormone excess or deficiencies.

Your management involves discussing with him the possibility of a persistent visual field deficit as well as diplopia. However, you are always optimistic explaining the possibility of some improvement, knowing there are no rules and only time will tell his final outcome. Even if long term diplopia, you reassure him regarding prism correction or future strabismus surgery providing a solution. You try to be even more encouraging if his non-congruous field deficit remains, explaining he may be more likely to adapt and compensate over time versus a "denser" field deficit as found in occipital lobe etiologies.

Post surgery, you schedule follow-up visual fields every 4 months during the year which will hopefully show some resolution. He has been wearing a patch over his right eye eliminating diplopia, however, in 1 month you can consider adding prism correction in glasses if stable diplopia.

Differential Diagnoses and Rationale

- **Pituitary Adenoma with Suprasellar Extension:** Detected on MRI, compressing the right optic tract and VI cranial nerve creating a corresponding visual field deficit and horizontal diplopia. This diagnosis required urgent neurosurgical intervention.
- **Cranial Diabetic Neuropathy:** Common in patients with longstanding diabetes, characterized by microvascular ischemia affecting the cranial nerves.
- **Giant Cell Arteritis/Temporal Arteritis:** Less likely given his lack of symptoms such as a temporal headache or tenderness, scalp tenderness, and/or jaw claudication.
- **Hypertensive Crisis:** Possible etiology of acute cranial nerve palsies, but less likely provided well-controlled blood pressure and lack of associated retinopathy.

- **Multiple Sclerosis with VI Nerve Palsy:** Unlikely given his age and acute non-comitant presentation without other neurologic signs suggestive of demyelination.

Learning Points

- Identify clinical signs and symptoms of a VI cranial nerve (abducens nerve) palsy, which include horizontal diplopia and limited abduction of the affected eye.
- Understand the significance of a thorough medical history in patients presenting with diplopia. Conditions like diabetes, hypertension, and hyperlipidemia increase the risk of microvascular cranial nerve palsies and need to be factored into the diagnostic process.
- Appreciate the necessity of imaging studies such as MRI in identifying underlying causes of cranial nerve palsies, including masses, vascular anomalies, or demyelinating disease.
- Recognize management strategies for cranial diabetic neuropathy, which include optimizing blood glucose control and monitoring for spontaneous recovery, which often occurs over weeks to months. Understanding the natural course helps in setting individual expectations.

Questions

Why is it important to order or obtain an emergent MRI in cases of diplopia in diabetes?

So to quickly rule-out compressive or structural sources which can also create a cranial nerve palsy, ensuring more ominous underlying conditions are not overlooked.

What are some characteristic symptoms of cranial diabetic neuropathy?

Cranial diabetic neuropathy typically presents with sudden onset diplopia, often without associated pain due to microvascular ischemia affecting a specific cranial nerve. VIn palsies are particularly common in individuals with diabetes.

Why should giant cell arteritis be considered in older patients with sudden visual symptoms or diplopia?

Giant cell arteritis can induce an "arteritic" ischemic optic neuropathy (AION), leading to painful sudden vision loss and/or diplopia. It is equally important to investigate due to high risk of stroke if left untreated.

How can a pituitary adenoma create a cranial nerve palsy and diplopia?

It can potentially occur with suprasellar extension compressing a nearby cranial nerve, such as the VI nerve leading to horizontal diplopia.

What is the significance of his mild, intermittent headaches?

Headaches may indicate increased intracranial pressure or other neurologic conditions that warrant further investigation. In his case, an atypical pituitary adenoma was discovered.

Thank You

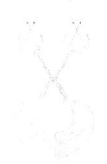

Thank you for taking time to read through some examples of what I believe to be fascinating and high-yield clinical scenarios. I hope the cases I've shared have not only helped enhance your clinical knowledge but have also provided practical concepts you can use in daily practice.

I understand the challenges you face in diagnosing and managing patients with overlapping ocular, medical, and neurologic conditions. My goal with this book is to help bridge those gaps, offering you detailed real-world scenarios highlighting the importance of a comprehensive and multidisciplinary approach to patient care.

Each case reflects the complexities and nuances taken from real clinical practice. From subtle signs of optic neuritis, to the multifaceted presentations of medical conditions affecting vision, these scenarios underscore the importance of thorough history-taking, review of systems, detailed physical examinations, strategic use of diagnostic tools, and proper management.

I especially hope you found the discussions and management sections insightful, helping you think more critically and expansively about differential diagnoses and management choices. The learning points and questions at the end of each case are intended to reinforce key concepts and encourage deeper thinking.

Applying these concepts into your practice can significantly improve patient outcomes, ensuring you are not only addressing the symptoms but also uncovering and managing underlying causes. And remember, our role in medicine and healthcare is not to just treat, but to educate and empower our patients guiding them through their journey with expertise and compassion.

Thank you once again for reading. I truly hope the knowledge and concepts you've gained from this book will enhance your practice and provide real-world benefits for your patients. Cheers to continued learning and excellence in taking care of people!

Warm regards,

- John

June 16, 2024

Resources

American Optometric Association (AOA)

Website: aoa.org

Provides information on eye care, optometric practice, and continuing education for optometrists.

American Academy of Ophthalmology (AAO)

Website: aao.org

Offers extensive resources on eye health, clinical guidelines, and educational materials for ophthalmologists and optometrists.

Johns Hopkins Medicine: Wilmer Eye Institute

Website: hopkinsmedicine.org/wilmer

Provides extensive resources on eye conditions, treatments, and research.

National Eye Institute (NEI)

Website: nei.nih.gov

A division of the NIH that offers comprehensive information on eye diseases, clinical research, and patient resources.

American Academy of Family Physicians (AAFP)

Website: aafp.org

Provides resources and guidelines for family physicians, including sections on eye health and neurologic conditions.

National Institute of Neurological Disorders and Stroke (NINDS)

Website: ninds.nih.gov

A division of the NIH that offers information on neurologic conditions, clinical trials, and research updates.

Mayo Clinic

Website: mayoclinic.org

Offers detailed articles on a wide range of medical conditions, including those affecting vision and neurologic health.

UpToDate

Website: uptodate.com

A clinical decision support resource used by healthcare professionals to provide evidence-based information on medical topics.

PubMed

Website: pubmed.ncbi.nlm.nih.gov

A free search engine accessing primarily the MEDLINE database of references and abstracts on life sciences and biomedical topics.

WebMD

Website: webmd.com

Offers patient-friendly information on a wide range of health issues, including eye and neurologic conditions.

Ophthalmic Terminology and Concepts

Afferent Pupillary Defect (APD): A condition indicating an abnormality in the sensory (afferent) pathway of the optic nerve, detected by the swinging flashlight test. The affected eye shows a diminished or absent pupillary response compared to the healthy eye.

Amaurosis Fugax: Transient monocular vision loss due to temporary ischemia of the retina or optic nerve, often caused by emboli originating from atherosclerotic plaques in the carotid artery.

Amblyopia: A neurodevelopmental disorder characterized by reduced visual acuity in one eye due to abnormal visual experience during early childhood, often without an identifiable ocular pathology.

Anisocoria: A condition characterized by unequal pupil sizes, which can be physiological or indicative of underlying neurological conditions.

Anterior Ischemic Optic Neuropathy (AION): A condition characterized by sudden, painless vision loss due to interrupted blood flow to the optic nerve head, which can be arteritic (linked to giant cell arteritis) or non-arteritic (often associated with vascular risk factors).

Anterior Uveitis: Inflammation of the uveal tract, specifically the iris and ciliary body, causing pain, redness, photophobia, and blurred vision. It can be associated with systemic diseases like HLA-B27-associated conditions.

Arteriovenous Malformation (AVM): An abnormal tangle of blood vessels connecting arteries and veins, which can disrupt normal blood flow and oxygen circulation. AVMs can occur in the brain and lead to intracranial hemorrhage, seizures, and neurological deficits.

Atherosclerotic Plaque: Accumulations of fatty deposits, cholesterol, and other substances in the arterial walls, leading to narrowing and potential blockage of blood vessels.

Autonomic Dysfunction: A condition where the autonomic nervous system (ANS) fails to regulate the body's involuntary functions properly, leading to symptoms such as orthostatic hypotension, syncope, and other cardiovascular anomalies.

Bitemporal Hemianopia: A visual field defect affecting the outer (temporal) halves of both visual fields, often indicative of a lesion at the optic chiasm, commonly caused by pituitary tumors or other midline brain structures.

Blepharitis: Inflammation of the eyelids, typically involving the margins where eyelashes grow. It can cause redness, irritation, itching, and flaking of the skin around the eyes.

Carotid Artery Stenosis: Narrowing of the carotid arteries, usually due to atherosclerosis, which can reduce blood flow to the brain and increase the risk of transient ischemic attacks (TIAs) and strokes.

Cavernous Sinus Thrombosis: A rare but serious condition involving the formation of a blood clot within the cavernous sinus, a large vein at the base of the brain, which can lead to severe neurological deficits and requires immediate medical intervention.

Central Retinal Artery Occlusion (CRAO): A sudden blockage of the central retinal artery, leading to acute, painless vision loss in the affected eye, often described as a "cherry-red spot" on the retina during examination.

Central Retinal Vein Occlusion (CRVO): Blockage of the central retinal vein, leading to retinal hemorrhages, macular edema, and potential vision loss, often associated with systemic conditions like hypertension and diabetes.

Cerebral Aneurysm: A weak or thin spot on a blood vessel in the brain that balloons and fills with blood. It can rupture, leading to subarachnoid hemorrhage, which is a life-threatening condition.

Cerebral Venous Sinus Thrombosis (CVST): Thrombosis in the dural venous sinuses, which can lead to increased intracranial pressure, headaches, seizures, and focal neurological deficits. Often associated with hypercoagulable states or infections.

Chiasmal Syndrome: A group of signs and symptoms resulting from a lesion at the optic chiasm, typically characterized by bitemporal hemianopia, optic atrophy, and potentially endocrine dysfunction if the pituitary gland is involved.

Choroidal Neovascularization (CNV): The growth of new blood vessels in the choroid layer of the eye, often associated with age-related macular degeneration (AMD), leading to vision loss.

Chorioretinitis: Inflammation of the choroid and retina, often due to infections, autoimmune diseases, or idiopathic causes, leading to vision loss if untreated.

Cluster Headaches: A type of primary headache disorder characterized by severe, unilateral pain typically around the eye, occurring in clusters over weeks or months, often associated with autonomic symptoms such as ptosis, lacrimation, and nasal congestion.

Coloboma: A congenital defect resulting in missing tissue in structures such as the iris, retina, choroid, or optic nerve, leading to visual field defects and other vision problems.

Cranial Nerve III (Oculomotor Nerve): Controls most of the eye's movements, including constriction of the pupil and maintaining an open eyelid via the levator palpebrae superioris muscle. Damage can result in ptosis, mydriasis, and eye movement abnormalities.

Cranial Nerve III Palsy: Dysfunction of the oculomotor nerve leading to ptosis, diplopia, and anisocoria due to impaired movement of the superior, inferior, and medial rectus muscles, as well as the levator palpebrae and pupillary sphincter muscles.

Cranial Nerve IV (Trochlear Nerve): Innervates the superior oblique muscle, which controls downward and inward eye movement. Lesions result in vertical diplopia and difficulty in reading or descending stairs.

Cranial Nerve IV Palsy: A condition resulting from dysfunction of the trochlear nerve, leading to vertical or oblique diplopia and difficulty in reading or descending stairs due to impaired movement of the superior oblique muscle.

Cranial Nerve V (Trigeminal Nerve): Provides sensory information from the face and motor innervation to the muscles of mastication. It has three branches: ophthalmic (V1), maxillary (V2), and mandibular (V3). Damage can cause facial pain or loss of sensation.

Cranial Nerve VI (Abducens Nerve): Innervates the lateral rectus muscle, responsible for abduction of the eye. Damage leads to horizontal diplopia and an inability to move the eye outward.

Cranial Nerve VI Palsy: A condition resulting from dysfunction of the abducens nerve, leading to horizontal diplopia and an inability to move the eye outward due to impaired function of the lateral rectus muscle.

Cranial Nerve VII (Facial Nerve): Controls the muscles of facial expression, provides taste sensations from the anterior two-thirds of the tongue, and supplies parasympathetic fibers to the lacrimal and salivary glands. Damage can cause facial paralysis, loss of taste, and dry eye or mouth.

Cranial Nerve Palsy: Dysfunction of one of the cranial nerves leading to deficits in sensory or motor function. Common examples include III, IV, and VI nerve palsies, resulting in ocular motor dysfunction and diplopia.

Demyelinating Disease: Disorders characterized by damage to the myelin sheath of neurons, such as multiple sclerosis (MS). These diseases lead to impaired signal transmission along nerve fibers and present with a variety of neurological symptoms.

Diabetic Retinopathy: A microvascular complication of diabetes mellitus characterized by damage to the blood vessels of the retina, leading to retinal hemorrhages, microaneurysms, hard exudates, and potentially macular edema or proliferative changes with neovascularization.

Diplopia: The perception of two images of a single object. It can be binocular (present when both eyes are open) or monocular (present in one eye even when the other is closed).

Disc Edema: Swelling of the optic disc, often indicative of increased intracranial pressure or optic nerve pathology, which can lead to vision loss if untreated.

Disciform Scar: A scar formation in the macula resulting from the end stage of wet age-related macular degeneration, leading to permanent central vision loss.

Dysautonomia: A disorder of the autonomic nervous system, affecting bodily functions such as heart rate, blood pressure, digestion, and temperature regulation.

Dry Eye Syndrome: A condition characterized by insufficient tear production or poor tear quality, leading to eye discomfort, visual disturbances, and an increased risk of ocular surface damage.

Embolic Stroke: A type of ischemic stroke caused by an embolus traveling from another part of the body, often the heart, blocking a cerebral artery and causing brain tissue damage.

Endophthalmitis: A severe, sight-threatening inflammation of the interior of the eye, often due to infection following surgery, trauma, or intraocular injections.

Epiretinal Membrane (ERM): A fibrocellular tissue that can form on the surface of the retina, leading to visual distortion and decreased visual acuity. It often requires surgical removal.

Epileptic Aura: A sensory, motor, or psychic phenomenon that precedes the onset of a seizure, providing a warning sign. Auras can include visual, auditory, olfactory, or gustatory hallucinations, as well as feelings of déjà vu or fear.

Esotropia: A form of strabismus where one or both eyes turn inward, leading to crossed eyes. It can be constant or intermittent and often requires corrective surgery or vision therapy.

Flashes and Floaters: Visual disturbances often caused by posterior vitreous detachment or retinal tears. Flashes are perceived as brief bursts of light, while floaters appear as small moving spots or threads in the visual field.

Gaze-Evoked Amaurosis: Transient loss of vision that occurs with certain eye movements, often indicative of optic nerve sheath meningioma or other lesions that exert pressure on the optic nerve during gaze shifts.

Giant Cell Arteritis (GCA): An inflammatory vasculitis affecting large and medium-sized arteries, primarily affecting the temporal arteries. It presents with headache, jaw claudication, visual disturbances, and an elevated erythrocyte sedimentation rate (ESR). Immediate treatment is necessary to prevent blindness.

Horner's Syndrome: A neurological disorder characterized by ptosis, miosis, and anhidrosis due to disruption of the sympathetic nerves supplying the eye and surrounding facial structures. It can result from lesions at various points along the sympathetic pathway.

Hyperemia: Increased blood flow in the blood vessels, leading to redness of the eye. It can be caused by inflammation, infection, or irritation.

Hypertensive Retinopathy: Retinal vascular changes due to chronic hypertension, characterized by arteriolar narrowing, arteriovenous nicking, retinal hemorrhages, exudates, and in severe cases, papilledema.

Idiopathic Intracranial Hypertension (IIH): A condition characterized by increased intracranial pressure without an apparent cause, leading to symptoms such as headache, transient visual obscurations, and papilledema. Often seen in young, obese women.

Intracranial Mass Effect: The pressure exerted by a mass lesion, such as a tumor, abscess, or hematoma, within the cranial cavity, leading to displacement of brain structures and potentially herniation.

Ischemic Optic Neuropathy (ION): An ischemic event leading to damage of the optic nerve, which can be arteritic (associated with conditions like giant cell arteritis) or non-arteritic (typically related to cardiovascular risk factors).

Juvenile Idiopathic Arthritis (JIA): An autoimmune disorder in children causing persistent joint inflammation. It can be associated with uveitis, leading to ocular complications and vision loss.

Keratoconus: A progressive eye disease where the cornea thins and bulges into a cone shape, leading to distorted vision. It often requires special contact lenses or corneal cross-linking.

Lateral Geniculate Nucleus (LGN): A relay center in the thalamus for the visual pathway, receiving input from the retinal ganglion cells and sending information to the visual cortex.

Lumbar Puncture: A diagnostic and therapeutic procedure involving the insertion of a needle into the subarachnoid space of the lumbar spine to collect cerebrospinal fluid (CSF) for analysis or to reduce intracranial pressure.

Macular Edema: Swelling or thickening of the macula, the central area of the retina responsible for detailed vision. It can result from diabetic retinopathy, retinal vein occlusion, or inflammation.

Marcus Gunn Pupil: An abnormal pupillary response where there is a relative afferent pupillary defect (RAPD). When light is shone in the affected eye, both pupils dilate instead of constricting due to an asymmetry in the afferent input between the two eyes.

Metamorphopsia: Visual distortion where straight lines appear wavy or curved, commonly associated with macular diseases such as age-related macular degeneration or epiretinal membranes.

Migraine with Aura: A subtype of migraine headache characterized by transient neurological symptoms such as visual disturbances, sensory phenomena, or speech difficulties that precede the headache phase.

Mononeuritis Multiplex: A condition involving damage to two or more separate nerve areas, often due to systemic diseases such as diabetes mellitus, vasculitis, or infections. It presents with asymmetric motor and sensory deficits.

Myasthenia Gravis: An autoimmune neuromuscular disorder characterized by weakness and rapid fatigue of voluntary muscles, due to autoantibodies against acetylcholine receptors at the neuromuscular junction.

Neovascular Glaucoma: A severe form of glaucoma characterized by the growth of new, abnormal blood vessels on the iris and over the drainage angle, leading to increased intraocular pressure and vision loss.

Neovascularization: The formation of new blood vessels, often occurring in response to ischemia. It can be seen in conditions like diabetic retinopathy and neovascular age-related macular degeneration, potentially leading to vision-threatening complications.

Neurogenic Claudication: A symptom of lumbar spinal stenosis characterized by pain and discomfort in the lower back, buttocks, and legs that is exacerbated by walking or standing and relieved by sitting or leaning forward.

Neuroprotection: Strategies aimed at preserving neuronal structure and function in the face of insult or injury, particularly in diseases like glaucoma, where optic nerve protection is critical.

Non-Arteritic Anterior Ischemic Optic Neuropathy (NAION): A condition characterized by sudden, painless vision loss in one eye due to infarction of the optic nerve head, typically associated with systemic vascular risk factors.

Nystagmus: Involuntary, rapid, and repetitive movement of the eyes. It can be congenital or acquired and may be associated with other neurological or ocular conditions.

Occipital Lobe Infarction: A stroke affecting the occipital lobe of the brain, which can lead to contralateral homonymous hemianopia, cortical blindness, or visual hallucinations.

Ocular Ischemic Syndrome: A condition caused by severe carotid artery stenosis or occlusion leading to reduced blood flow to the eye, resulting in symptoms such as visual loss, pain, and retinal findings like hemorrhages and neovascularization.

Ophthalmoplegia: Paralysis or weakness of one or more of the muscles that control eye movement, resulting in impaired movement of the eyes and potentially leading to diplopia and strabismus. It can be due to nerve damage, myasthenia gravis, or mitochondrial diseases.

Optic Neuritis: Inflammation of the optic nerve, often associated with demyelinating diseases such as multiple sclerosis. Presents with painful vision loss, particularly with eye movement, and can be retrobulbar or anterior.

Optical Coherence Tomography (OCT): A non-invasive imaging technique used to obtain high-resolution cross-sectional images of the retina, aiding in the diagnosis and monitoring of various ocular conditions, particularly retinal and optic nerve diseases.

Papilledema: Swelling of the optic disc due to increased intracranial pressure. It is a sign of significant intracranial pathology and warrants prompt evaluation to determine the underlying cause.

Papillitis: Inflammation of the optic nerve head, presenting with disc edema and often associated with optic neuritis. It is distinguished from retrobulbar neuritis, where the inflammation is behind the eye and the optic disc appears normal.

Paraneoplastic Syndromes: A group of rare disorders triggered by an abnormal immune response to a neoplasm. These syndromes can affect various organ systems, including the nervous system, leading to conditions such as Lambert-Eaton myasthenic syndrome and opsoclonus-myoclonus syndrome.

Photopsia: The sensation of seeing flashes of light, often indicative of retinal detachment, migraine aura, or other ocular or neurological conditions.

Posterior Capsular Opacification (PCO): A common complication of cataract surgery where the posterior capsule becomes opacified, leading to vision loss. It is typically treated with a YAG laser capsulotomy.

Posterior Vitreous Detachment (PVD): The separation of the vitreous gel from the retina, a common age-related change that can lead to floaters and flashes, and sometimes retinal tears.

Postural Orthostatic Tachycardia Syndrome (POTS): A condition characterized by excessive heart rate increase upon standing, leading to symptoms such as lightheadedness, palpitations, and occasionally syncope. It is often a form of autonomic dysfunction.

Prolactinoma: A benign pituitary adenoma that produces prolactin, leading to symptoms such as galactorrhea, amenorrhea, and hypogonadism. It can also cause visual disturbances if it compresses the optic chiasm.

Pseudotumor Cerebri (Idiopathic Intracranial Hypertension): A condition characterized by increased intracranial pressure without an apparent cause, leading to symptoms such as headache, transient visual obscurations, and papilledema.

Relative Afferent Pupillary Defect (RAPD): A clinical finding indicative of an asymmetry in optic nerve function between the two eyes. It is typically assessed using the swinging flashlight test and is a hallmark of optic neuropathy.

Retinal Detachment: A medical emergency where the retina separates from the underlying supportive tissue, leading to potential permanent vision loss if not promptly treated. Symptoms include the sudden appearance of floaters, flashes of light, and a shadow or curtain over part of the visual field.

Retinal Nerve Fiber Layer (RNFL): The layer of the retina composed of the axons of the retinal ganglion cells. RNFL thinning, detected by optical coherence tomography (OCT), is an important diagnostic marker for glaucomatous damage and other optic neuropathies.

Retinal Vein Occlusion (RVO): Blockage of the retinal veins, leading to sudden painless vision loss, retinal hemorrhages, and macular edema. It is associated with systemic vascular conditions such as hypertension and diabetes.

Retinitis Pigmentosa (RP): A group of inherited disorders characterized by progressive peripheral vision loss and night blindness due to the degeneration of the retinal photoreceptor cells.

Saccadic Intrusions: Abnormal, rapid eye movements that interrupt smooth pursuit or fixation, often seen in conditions affecting the cerebellum or its connections, such as multiple sclerosis or neurodegenerative diseases.

Scintillating Scotoma: A visual aura often seen in migraines, characterized by shimmering or flickering lights in the visual field, often preceding the headache phase of a migraine.

Sixth Nerve Palsy: Paralysis of the abducens nerve, leading to an inability to abduct the eye. It can result from increased intracranial pressure, trauma, ischemia, or neoplastic processes affecting the nerve along its course.

Skew Deviation: A vertical misalignment of the eyes due to disruption of the vestibular pathways, often indicative of brainstem or cerebellar lesions. It is typically associated with other signs of central nervous system dysfunction.

Strabismus: A condition where the eyes do not properly align with each other when looking at an object, leading to double vision or amblyopia if untreated. It can be caused by muscle imbalance or nerve dysfunction.

Subarachnoid Hemorrhage: Bleeding into the subarachnoid space, often due to a ruptured aneurysm or arteriovenous malformation. It presents with sudden, severe headache, often described as the "worst headache of my life," and can lead to neurological deficits and increased intracranial pressure.

Temporal Arteritis (Giant Cell Arteritis): An inflammatory disease of the large and medium-sized arteries, primarily affecting the temporal arteries. It presents with headache, jaw claudication, visual disturbances, and an elevated erythrocyte sedimentation rate (ESR). Immediate treatment is necessary to prevent blindness.

Tonic Pupil (Adie's Pupil): A dilated pupil with poor or absent light response and slow, tonic constriction to near effort, often due to damage to the post-ganglionic parasympathetic fibers innervating the pupillary sphincter muscle.

Trigeminal Autonomic Cephalalgias (TACs): A group of primary headache disorders characterized by unilateral headache with ipsilateral cranial autonomic symptoms. Includes conditions such as cluster headache, paroxysmal hemicrania, and SUNCT syndrome.

Trigeminal Neuralgia: A chronic pain condition affecting the trigeminal nerve, characterized by intense, episodic facial pain. It is often triggered by routine activities such as eating or speaking and can be highly debilitating.

Vagus Nerve Dysfunction: Dysfunction of the tenth cranial nerve, which can lead to a variety of symptoms including syncope, bradycardia, gastrointestinal dysmotility, and vocal cord paralysis.

Vascular Endothelial Growth Factor (VEGF): A protein that promotes the growth of new blood vessels. Overexpression can lead to diseases such as diabetic retinopathy and age-related macular degeneration, where abnormal blood vessel growth causes vision loss.

Vertebrobasilar Insufficiency: A condition resulting from reduced blood flow in the vertebrobasilar arterial system, leading to symptoms like vertigo, dizziness, visual disturbances, and syncope. It is commonly due to atherosclerotic disease affecting the vertebral and basilar arteries.

About the Author

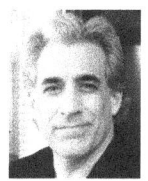

With 27 years on the private practice front lines as an optometric physician prior to earning his MD, Dr. Martinelli brings years of extensive clinical experience, combined with medicine, providing rare insight and guidance in the art of patient management.

He offers not theory, but high-yield clinical knowledge to help build the practice you deserve simply by taking proper care of people, who also happen to be your patients.

Dr. Martinelli is a graduate of St. George's University School of Medicine, Pennsylvania College of Optometry, and Washington & Jefferson College. He is a physician member of the American Medical Association (AMA), American Optometric Association (AOA), and Fellow of the American Academy of Optometry (FAAO).

His clinical articles have been featured over the years in various publications. He very much enjoys teaching, and for more than a decade taught countless students in his practice as a preceptor in ocular disease for the Pennsylvania College of Optometry.

Dr. Martinelli has spoken for Alcon and Allergan, as well as nationally and internationally with topics involving medical eye care, glaucoma, and refractive surgery such as LASIK.

He continues to actively see patients daily in private practice.

Ophthalmic Physician Website

www.ingramcontent.com/pod-product-compliance
Lightning Source LLC
Chambersburg PA
CBHW051142120626
46547CB00012B/913